Mosby's Advanced
Pharmacy Technician

MOSBY'S®
ADVANCED PHARMACY TECHNICIAN

KAREN DAVIS, AAHCA, BHS, CPhT
INSTRUCTOR, PHARMACY TECHNICIAN PROGRAM
PENN FOSTER CAREER COLLEGE
SCRANTON, PENNSYLVANIA;
PRESIDENT AND OWNER
ACCREDITATION ALLIANCE CONSULTING SERVICES
SOCIETY FOR THE EDUCATION OF PHARMACY TECHNICIANS
(SEPhT)
LYONS, GEORGIA

ELSEVIER

Elsevier
3251 Riverport Lane
St. Louis, Missouri 63043

MOSBY'S ADVANCED PHARMACY TECHNICIAN, FIRST EDITION   ISBN: 978-0-323-76141-3

Notice

Practitioners and researchers must always rely on their own experience and knowledge in evaluating and using any information, methods, compounds or experiments described herein. Because of rapid advances in the medical sciences, in particular, independent verification of diagnoses and drug dosages should be made. To the fullest extent of the law, no responsibility is assumed by Elsevier, authors, editors or contributors for any injury and/or damage to persons or property as a matter of products liability, negligence or otherwise, or from any use or operation of any methods, products, instructions, or ideas contained in the material herein.

International Standard Book Number: 978-0-323761413

Content Director: Kristin Wilhelm
Content Development Manager: Laurie Gower
Content Development Specialist: Brooke Kannady
Publishing Services Manager: Shereen Jameel
Project Manager: Aparna Venkatachalam
Design Director: Bridget Hoette

Printed in China

Last digit is the print number: 9   8   7   6   5   4   3   2   1

Working together to grow libraries in developing countries

www.elsevier.com • www.bookaid.org

List of Reviewers

Dina H. Adams, PharmD, RPh
Department Chair
Pharmacy Technology
Fayetteville Technical Community College
Fayetteville, North Carolina

Christine A. Cline-Dalman, BFA, CPhT
Georgia Board of Pharmacy, PTCB Certified
Director of Education and Training
Institute for Wellness and Education
Private education firm—pharmacy and patient
Woodstock, Georgia

Kendra N. Johnson, CPhT
PTCB Certified Pharmacy Technician
Allied Health Program Coordinator Pharmacy
    Technician Program
Adult Education—Pharmacy Technician
Pickaway Ross Career & Technology Center
Chillicothe, Ohio

**Wendy M. Lane, RPhT, CPhT, A.S, HIPAA Certified,
    ServSafe Certified**
Pending Certifications MTM for Diabetes and MTM
Pharmacy Technician Instructor
Career Transition Training
Westover Job Corps
Chicopee, Massachusetts

James J. Mizner Jr., MBA, BS, RPh
Panacea Solutions Consulting
Reston, Virginia

Lori J. Stepp, BSE, CPhT
Academic Program Director
Pharmacy Technician Program
Greenville Technical College
Greenville, South Carolina

Preface

With the evolution of the healthcare system, particularly toward a patient-centered model, the technician's role is expanding and providing advanced opportunities that have an integral role in the profession. In the past, technicians had limited functions, and there were restrictions on many common tasks performed in the traditional pharmacy. Today's modern pharmacy incorporates additional responsibilities and a greater leadership role for technicians who seek specialty certifications and advanced training. American Society of Health-System Pharmacists (ASHP)/ Accreditation Council for Pharmacy Education (ACPE) technician training programs were revised in 2019 to include programs for the entry and advanced levels, and the Pharmacy Technician Certification Board (PTCB) added several specialty certifications for certified pharmacy technicians (CPhTs) wishing to specialize in specific areas.

As a practicing technician and educator for over 35 years, I wanted to provide information for practicing technicians to challenge them to step outside of their comfort zones and empower them to take on larger responsibilities and advanced roles in their careers. This will improve patient outcomes and help streamline our healthcare for the future.

Pharmacy technicians currently enrolled in advanced technician programs should be encouraged to see the profession as offering a career ladder that can provide a lifelong learning experience in many different areas. Career technicians with experience in the profession can use the information provided to seek a specialty area and become certified or advanced to allow them to advance into areas offered within their current practice environment. Being a team member of a successful pharmacy is rewarding and creates a blended team and added recognition.

Today's pharmacist role is clinical, and as the population continues to age, there will be an increase in prescriptions and the need for high-quality counseling. As pharmacists become more involved as providers, more of the day-to-day tasks in the pharmacy will be left to trained technicians. Pharmacists must have confidence in the abilities of technicians because this is critical in providing patient-centered care while competing in the current healthcare model.

The focus on medication adherence requires a systematic approach with effective communication, monitoring, and follow-up analysis of data. The tasks can be performed by a trained technician in an advanced role and serve to provide affordable and efficient services for patients.

New Key Features

- **Built from ASHP and PTCB standards** to match coverage required in advanced-level pharmacy technician programs and focus on the five advanced-level certificate programs to meet the new advanced certified pharmacy technician (CPhT-Adv) credential
- **Comprehensive coverage** of tech check tech, medication history and reconciliation, controlled substance diversion prevention, billing and reimbursement, hazardous drug management, and a variety of management and leadership topics to help build a supervisory skill set
- **Step-by-step illustrated procedures** with rationales for key skills and competencies
- **Study practice,** including review questions at the end of each chapter, exam-review appendix with sample questions, and review questions online
- **Emphasis on real-world problem solving** with chapter case studies
- *Tech Notes* **and** *Tech Alerts* with practical tips for on-the-job accuracy and efficiency
- **Robust companion website** with resources to save instructors course-preparation time and help students study and prepare for class examinations

Evolve Instructor Resources
- TEACH Instructor Resource Manual
  - Lesson plans mapping content to learning objectives
  - PowerPoint slides with talking points
  - Student handouts
  - Answer keys
- Test bank—500 questions, each with answer, rationales for correct and incorrect responses, cognitive leveling, and mapping to chapter objectives and exam blueprints
- Image collection
- Competency skill checklists
- Accreditation mapping guides

Evolve Student Resources
- Chapter practice quizzes
- Mock certification exam

By using the content and practice questions included, the reader can prepare for specialty exams and the CPhT-Adv exam. Subject areas include opportunities for advanced roles and descriptions of the tasks involved that can be used to advance through career ladders.

Dedication

I would like to thank my husband who has always supported and encouraged me to think big and never be afraid to try. I would also like to say thank you to Jennifer Janson and Kristin Wilhelm who both gave me many opportunities to grow as an author and help to advance the pharmacy technician career. This book has been a vision of mine for many years and I encourage technicians to always look for advancements and plan for a life long career in pharmacy.

Contents

Current and Expanding Role of the Pharmacy Technician

1

Learning Objectives

1. Discuss the changes in evolving role of the pharmacy technician.
2. List organizations associated with advancing the technician's role and responsibilities.
3. Identify the national certifications available to the technician.
4. Explain the ways advanced technician roles play a part in patient safety.

Key Terms

Accreditation Council for Pharmacy Education (ACPE) Organization that provides continuing education for pharmacy practitioners.

Accrediting Bureau of Health Education Schools (ABHES) Nonprofit, independent accrediting agency founded in 1969.

American Society of Health-System Pharmacists (ASHP) Organization whose mission is to support pharmacy professionals and promote patient medication safety.

ASHP/ACPE A collaboration between the American Society of Health-System Pharmacists and the Accreditation Council for Pharmacy Education.

Board of pharmacy (BOP) State agency responsible for licensing, registration, and regulating the responsibilities of pharmacists and technicians.

Certification Indicates successful completion a certain level of achievement through passing a competency-based exam.

Certified pharmacy technician (CPhT) A technician who has successfully passed the national certification exam.

ExCPT A national exam provided by the National Healthcare Association for certification of technicians.

Licensure Indicates that an individual has achieved a minimum level of competency.

National Association of Boards of Pharmacy (NABP) Nonprofit association that protects public health by assisting its member boards of pharmacy and offers programs that promote safe pharmacy practices for the benefit of consumers.

National Healthcare Association (NHA) Organization that offers a certification for pharmacy technicians through the Institute for Certification of Pharmacy Technicians.

Pharmacy Technician Accreditation Commission (PTAC) Combination of the American Society of Health-System Pharmacists and the Accreditation Council for Pharmacy Education to form the accreditation organization for technician training accreditation.

Pharmacy Technician Certification Board (PTCB) Organization that offers national certification of pharmacy technicians (CPhT).

Pharmacy Technician Certification Exam (PTCE) A national exam offered by the Pharmacy Technician Certification Board for the certification of technicians.

Registration Act of maintaining a list of practitioners; usually requires a background check.

INTRODUCTION

The field of pharmacy has evolved significantly over the years (Fig. 1.1). What began as a "compounder"—whom we know as a *pharmacist* today—an individual who prepared what a physician ordered by mixing herbs or using other natural remedies, evolved into a highly scientific and complicated process. Apothecaries were early pharmacies where pharmacists took on the role of dispensing medications when physicians began to diagnose diseases and perform surgeries. During the Civil War and other conflicts, advancements in medicine exploded as a result of the necessity of wound care and the aim of halting the spread of disease (Fig. 1.2).

The early pharmacy technician was often referred to as a *clerk* and generally was an assistant to the pharmacist, who possessed the necessary education and training. Because a clerk was an untrained person participating in the role of dispensing medications, it became quite evident early on that this was not the best way to provide the safest care or correct medication for a patient. Simple clerk or assistant duties included packaging, stocking, delivery, and basic accounting procedures and money transactions.

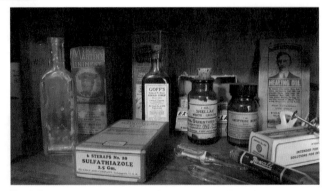

Fig. 1.1 Old medical collection. (Courtesy Karen Davis.)

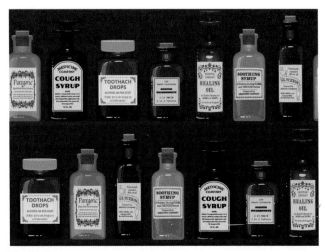

Fig. 1.2 Medicines that may have been available in an old apothecary. (Copyright © iStock.com/Sveta_Aho.)

CURRENT TECHNICIAN RESPONSIBILITIES

Technicians today work in a variety of settings. In each facility, there are basic responsibilities based on the facility policies and the state **board of pharmacy (BOP)** regulations. Each facility is allowed to create specific levels for technicians with specific job descriptions, but these must stay within the guidelines of the state BOP regulations for technicians. According to the **Pharmacy Technician Certification Board (PTCB)**, common responsibilities of pharmacy technicians across the country include the following:
- Receiving prescription requests
- Counting tablets and labeling bottles
- Maintaining patient profiles
- Submitting prescription claims
- Performing administrative functions, such as answering phones, stocking shelves, and operating cash registers (Fig. 1.3)

ADVANCED ROLES OF PHARMACY TECHNICIANS

As our understanding of the human body has increased, so have the treatment options—including the development of new pharmaceuticals. This means pharmacies are dispensing more medications, while more of the

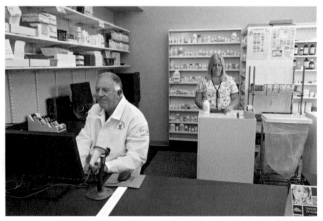

Fig. 1.3 Pharmacy technicians are assigned to designated spots for efficient workflow. (From Davis, K., & Guerra, A. [2019]. *Mosby's pharmacy technician* [5th ed.]. St. Louis, MO: Elsevier.)

pharmacist's time is being spent collaborating with other healthcare providers on patient care. Pharmacists now partner with physicians on drug dosing and patient consultations; they are part of team approach to the patient's overall health and disease management. Disease management and collaborative care are now part of standard care, and a technician must be an integral part of that endeavor. The day-to-day tasks that technicians are responsible for have changed, evolving from the role of a "drug clerk" or "assistant" who was trained on the job (OTJ) to a "technician," a skilled and technically advanced role that requires education and/or some type of verification of a basic knowledge of pharmacy. The dispensing and technical duties of the pharmacy are now performed by the technicians. In addition to the tasks listed previously for current technicians in most states, some of the advanced roles include the following:
- Inventory management
- Quality assurance
- Wellness and disease management support
- Medication reconciliation
- Patient advocate positions (performing tests, taking medical histories, immunizations)
- Compounding (sterile, nonsterile) of nonhazardous and hazardous medications (Fig. 1.4)

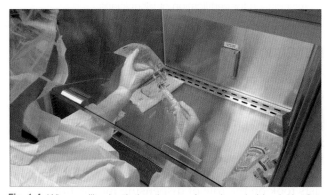

Fig. 1.4 When pulling back the plunger of a syringe, hold only the flat knob at the end to avoid compromising the barrel of the syringe if it will be used for more than one withdrawal. (Courtesy CriticalPoint, LLC, Totowa, New Jersey.)

ORGANIZATIONS INVOLVED IN TECHNICIAN TRAINING

In pharmacies across the country, the duties of the pharmacy technician are expanding. This has created challenges for an untrained workforce, and the need for skilled personnel has become more evident. This section discusses the organizations working to identify the requirements for training and the appropriate skill levels of pharmacy technicians.

PHARMACY TECHNICIAN CERTIFICATION BOARD

Beginning in 1995, the PTCB began offering a national certification exam known as the **Pharmacy Technician Certification Exam (PTCE)**. This was the first volunteer certification to provide a measure of base knowledge that was evaluated through a multiple-choice test. States and other national pharmacy organizations quickly began to recommend this exam as a way to ensure a technician had a basic knowledge of pharmacy practices. The nine areas that were covered consisted of basic tasks associated with pharmacy practice, such as pharmacology, law, compounding, medication safety, inventory, information systems, quality assurance, order entry, and billing. Effective January 1, 2020, the test

has four domains: medications, federal regulations, patient safety, and order entry and processing. To date, there is no educational requirement for taking this test; however, beginning in 2020, a technician who wishes to become a **certified pharmacy technician (CPhT)** will be required to be a graduate of a program accredited by the **ASHP/ACPE** or the **Accrediting Bureau of Health Education Schools (ABHES)** program to take the PTCE. Currently, all 50 states accept the PTCE as a board-approved certification test. In addition, the test outline has been updated, effective January 2020.

There are also specialty certifications available, such as the certified sterile processing technician (CSPT) credential and the advanced pharmacy technician (CPhT-Adv) certification, which was introduced in 2020 (Table 1.1).

NATIONAL HEALTH CAREER ASSOCIATION

The test provided by the **National Health career Association (NHA)** is the **ExCPT**, which is a multiple-choice exam. Areas covered include overview and laws, drugs and drug therapy, dispensing process, medication safety, and quality assurance. Some states do not recognize this test as a certification. See your local state BOP for the specific requirements in your state.

Table 1.1 Pharmacy Technician Certification Exam (PTCE) 2.0 to 3.0 Crosswalk

2019 PTCE KNOWLEDGE AREAS		2019 PTCE KNOWLEDGE AREA DESCRIPTION	2020 PTCE KNOWLEDGE AREAS	2020 PTCE KNOWLEDGE AREAS DESCRIPTION
Domain 1.0: Pharmacology for Technicians	1.1	Generic and brand names of pharmaceuticals	1.1	Generic names, brand names, and classifications of medications
	1.2	Therapeutic equivalence	1.2	Therapeutic equivalence
	1.3	Drug interactions (e.g., drug–disease, drug–drug, drug–dietary supplement, drug–over the counter [OTC], drug–laboratory, drug–nutrient)	1.3	Common and life-threatening drug interactions and contraindications (e.g., drug–disease, drug–drug, drug–dietary supplement, drug–laboratory, drug–nutrient)
	1.4	Strengths/dose, dosage forms, physical appearance, routes of administration, and duration of drug therapy	1.4	Strengths/dose, dosage forms, routes of administration, special handling and administration instructions, and duration of drug therapy
	1.5	Common and severe side or adverse effects, allergies, and therapeutic contraindications associated with medications	1.3	Common and life-threatening drug interactions and contraindications (e.g., drug–disease, drug–drug, drug–dietary supplement, drug–laboratory, drug–nutrient)
			1.5	Common and severe medication side effects, adverse effects, and allergies
	1.6	Dosage and indication of legend, OTC medications, herbal and dietary supplements	1.6	Indications of medications and dietary supplements
			1.8	Narrow therapeutic index (NTI) medications

Continued

Table 1.1 Pharmacy Technician Certification Exam (PTCE) 2.0 to 3.0 Crosswalk—cont'd

2019 PTCE KNOWLEDGE AREAS		2019 PTCE KNOWLEDGE AREA DESCRIPTION	2020 PTCE KNOWLEDGE AREAS	2020 PTCE KNOWLEDGE AREAS DESCRIPTION
Domain 2.0: Pharmacy Law and Regulations	2.1	Storage, handling, and disposal of hazardous substances and wastes (e.g., Material Safety Data Sheets [MSDSs])	2.1	Federal requirements for handling and disposal of nonhazardous, hazardous, and pharmaceutical substances and waste
	2.2	Hazardous substances exposure, prevention, and treatment (e.g., eyewash, spill kit, MSDS)	2.1	Federal requirements for handling and disposal of nonhazardous, hazardous, and pharmaceutical substances and waste
	2.3	Controlled substance transfer regulations (Drug Enforcement Agency [DEA])	2.2	Federal requirements for controlled substance prescriptions (i.e., new, refill, transfer) and DEA controlled substance schedules
	2.4	Controlled substance documentation requirements for receiving, ordering, returning, loss/theft, destruction (DEA)	2.3	Federal requirements for controlled substances (i.e., receiving, storing, ordering, labeling, dispensing, reverse distribution, take-back programs, loss or theft of, and destroying)
	2.5	Formula to verify the validity of a prescriber's DEA number (DEA)		
	2.6	Record keeping, documentation, and record retention (e.g., length of time prescriptions are maintained on file)	2.3	Federal requirements for controlled substances (i.e., receiving, storing, ordering, labeling, dispensing, reverse distribution, take-back programs, loss or theft of, and destroying)
	2.7	Restricted drug programs and related prescription-processing requirements (e.g., thalidomide, isotretinoin, clozapine)	2.4	Federal requirements for restricted drug programs and related medication processing (e.g., pseudoephedrine, risk evaluation and mitigation strategies [REMS])
	2.8	Professional standards related to data integrity, security, and confidentiality (e.g., Health Insurance Portability and Accountability Act [HIPAA], backing up and archiving)		
	2.9	Requirement for consultation (e.g., Omnibus Budget Reconciliation Act of 1990 [OBRA])		
	2.10	US Food and Drug Administration (FDA) recall classification	2.5	FDA recall requirements (e.g., medications, devices, supplies, supplements, classifications)
	2.11	Infection control standards (e.g., laminar airflow, clean room, handwashing, cleaning counting trays, countertop, and equipment) (Occupational Safety and Health Administration [OSHA], United States Pharmacopeia [USP 795] and 797)	3.6	Hygiene and cleaning standards (e.g., handwashing, personal protective equipment [PPE], cleaning counting trays, countertop, and equipment)
	2.12	Record keeping for repackaged and recalled products and supplies (The Joint Commission [TJC], boards of pharmacy [BOPs])		

Table 1.1 Pharmacy Technician Certification Exam (PTCE) 2.0 to 3.0 Crosswalk—cont'd

2019 PTCE KNOWLEDGE AREAS		2019 PTCE KNOWLEDGE AREA DESCRIPTION	2020 PTCE KNOWLEDGE AREAS	2020 PTCE KNOWLEDGE AREAS DESCRIPTION
	2.13	Professional standards regarding the roles and responsibilities of pharmacists, pharmacy technicians, and other pharmacy employees (TJC, BOP)		
	2.14	Reconciliation between state and federal laws and regulations		
	2.15	Facility, equipment, and supply requirements (e.g., space requirements, prescription file storage, cleanliness, reference materials) (TJC, USP, BOP)		
Domain 3.0: Sterile and Nonsterile Compounding	3.1	Infection control (e.g., handwashing, PPE)	3.6	Hygiene and cleaning standards (e.g., handwashing, PPE, cleaning counting trays, countertop, and equipment)
	3.2	Handling and disposal requirements (e.g., receptacles, waste streams)	2.1	Federal requirements for handling and disposal of nonhazardous, hazardous, and pharmaceutical substances and waste
	3.3	Documentation (e.g., batch preparation, compounding record)		
	3.4	Determine product stability (e.g., beyond-use dating, signs of incompatibility)	1.7	Drug stability (e.g., oral suspensions, insulin, reconstitutables, injectables, vaccinations)
			1.9	Physical and chemical incompatibilities related to nonsterile compounding and reconstitution
	3.5	Selection and use of equipment and supplies	4.3	Equipment/supplies required for drug administration (e.g., package size, unit dose, diabetic supplies, spacers, oral and injectable syringes)
	3.6	Sterile compounding processes		
	3.7	Nonsterile compounding processes	4.1	Procedures to compound nonsterile products (e.g., ointments, mixtures, liquids, emulsions, suppositories, enemas)
Domain 4.0: Medication Safety	4.1	Error-prevention strategies for data entry (e.g., prescription or medication order to correct patient)	3.2	Error-prevention strategies (e.g., prescription or medication order to correct patient, Tall Man lettering, separating inventory, leading and trailing zeros, barcode usage, limit use of error-prone abbreviations)
	4.2	Patient package insert and medication guide requirements (e.g., special directions and precautions)	2.4	Federal requirements for restricted drug programs and related medication processing (e.g., pseudoephedrine, REMS)
	4.3	Identify issues that require pharmacist intervention (e.g., drug utilization review [DUR], adverse drug event [ADE, OTC recommendation], therapeutic substitution, misuse, missed dose)	3.3	Issues that require pharmacist intervention (e.g., DUR, ADE, OTC recommendation, therapeutic substitution, misuse, adherence, postimmunization follow-up, allergies, drug interactions)

Continued

Table 1.1   Pharmacy Technician Certification Exam (PTCE) 2.0 to 3.0 Crosswalk—cont'd

2019 PTCE KNOWLEDGE AREAS		2019 PTCE KNOWLEDGE AREA DESCRIPTION	2020 PTCE KNOWLEDGE AREAS	2020 PTCE KNOWLEDGE AREAS DESCRIPTION
	4.4	Look-alike/sound-alike (LASA) medications	3.1	High-alert/high-risk medications and LASA medications
	4.5	High-alert/high-risk medications	3.1	High-alert/high-risk medications and LASA medications
	4.6	Common safety strategies (e.g., Tall Man lettering, separating inventory, leading and trailing zeros, limit use of error-prone abbreviations)	3.2	Error-prevention strategies (e.g., prescription or medication order to correct patient, Tall Man lettering, separating inventory, leading and trailing zeros, barcode usage, limit use of error-prone abbreviations)
Domain 5.0: Pharmacy Quality Assurance	5.1	Quality assurance practices for medication and inventory control systems (e.g., matching National Drug Code [NDC] number, barcode, data entry)	4.4	Lot numbers, expiration dates, and NDC numbers
	5.2	Infection control procedures and documentation (e.g., PPE, needle recapping)	3.6	Hygiene and cleaning standards (e.g., handwashing, PPE, cleaning counting trays, countertop, and equipment)
	5.3	Risk management guidelines and regulations (e.g., error-prevention strategies)	3.4	Event-reporting procedures (e.g., medication errors, adverse effects, and product integrity, MedWatch, near miss, root-cause analysis [RCA])
			3.5	Types of prescription errors (e.g., abnormal doses, early refill, incorrect quantity, incorrect patient, incorrect drug)
	5.4	Communication channels necessary to ensure appropriate follow-up and problem resolution (e.g., product recalls, shortages)	3.4	Event-reporting procedures (e.g., medication errors, adverse effects, and product integrity, MedWatch, near miss, RCA)
	5.5	Productivity, efficiency, and customer satisfaction measures		
Domain 6.0: Order Entry and Medication Filling Process	6.1	Order-entry process		
	6.2	Intake, interpretation, and data entry	4.2	Formulas, calculations, ratios, proportions, alligations, conversions, Sig codes (e.g., b.i.d., t.i.d., Roman numerals), abbreviations, medical terminology, and symbols for day's supply, quantity, dose, concentration, dilutions
	6.3	Calculate doses required	4.2	Formulas, calculations, ratios, proportions, alligations, conversions, Sig codes (e.g., b.i.d., t.i.d., Roman numerals), abbreviations, medical terminology, and symbols for day's supply, quantity, dose, concentration, dilutions
	6.4	Fill process (e.g., select appropriate product, apply special handling requirements, measure, and prepare product for final check)	4.3	Equipment/supplies required for drug administration (e.g., package size, unit dose, diabetic supplies, spacers, oral and injectable syringes)
	6.5	Labeling requirements (e.g., auxiliary and warning labels, expiration date, patient-specific information)		

Table 1.1 Pharmacy Technician Certification Exam (PTCE) 2.0 to 3.0 Crosswalk—cont'd

2019 PTCE KNOWLEDGE AREAS		2019 PTCE KNOWLEDGE AREA DESCRIPTION	2020 PTCE KNOWLEDGE AREAS	2020 PTCE KNOWLEDGE AREAS DESCRIPTION
	6.6	Packaging requirements (e.g., type of bags, syringes, glass, PVC, child resistant, light resistant)	1.10	Proper storage of medications (e.g., temperature ranges, light sensitivity, restricted access)
			4.3	Equipment/supplies required for drug administration (e.g., package size, unit dose, diabetic supplies, spacers, oral and injectable syringes)
	6.7	Dispensing process (e.g., validation, documentation, and distribution)		
Domain 7.0: Pharmacy Inventory Management	7.1	Function and application of NDC, lot numbers, and expiration dates	4.4	Lot numbers, expiration dates, and NDC numbers
	7.2	Formulary or approved/preferred product list		
	7.3	Ordering and receiving processes (e.g., maintain par levels, rotate stock)		
	7.4	Storage requirements (e.g., refrigeration, freezer, warmer)	1.10	Proper storage of medications (e.g., temperature ranges, light sensitivity, restricted access)
	7.5	Removal (e.g., recalls, returns, outdates, reverse distribution)	4.5	Procedures for identifying and returning dispensable, nondispensable, and expired medications and supplies (e.g., credit return, return to stock, reverse distribution)
Domain 8.0: Pharmacy Billing and Reimbursement	8.1	Reimbursement policies and plans (e.g., health maintenance organizations [HMOs], preferred provider organizations [PPOs], Centers for Medicare and Medicaid [CMS], private plans)		
	8.2	Third-party resolution (e.g., prior authorization, rejected claims, plan limitations)		
	8.3	Third-party reimbursement systems (e.g., pharmacy benefit manager [PBM], medication assistance programs, coupons, and self-pay)		
	8.4	Healthcare reimbursement systems (e.g., home health, long-term care, home infusion)		
	8.5	Coordination of benefits		
Domain 9.0: Pharmacy Information System Usage and Application	9.1	Pharmacy-related computer applications for documenting the dispensing of prescriptions or medication orders (e.g., maintaining the electronic medical record, patient adherence, risk factors, alcohol and drug use, drug allergies, side effects)		
	9.2	Databases, pharmacy computer applications, and documentation management (e.g., user access, drug database, interface, inventory report, usage reports, override reports, diversion reports)		

NATIONAL ASSOCIATION OF BOARDS OF PHARMACY

Pharmacy organizations such as the **National Association of Boards of Pharmacy (NABP)** have begun to work toward a consensus on national standards for training and credentialing of pharmacy technicians. The NABP was founded in 1904 and oversees the state BOPs. Each state has the autonomy to set its own rules and criteria for pharmacists and technicians to practice in that state.

 Tech Note

If a federal law and a state law differ, whichever is the strictest applies.

In 2009, the NABP's Task Force on Pharmacy Technicians Education and Training Programs met to discuss the future of pharmacy technicians. Following this meeting, the NABP recommended the state BOPs to register pharmacy technicians and require them to complete a technician training program. This is a recommendation, and each state can decide on its own rules based on the state's best interest.

STATE BOARDS OF PHARMACY

Each state has a BOP that regulates the practice of pharmacy in that state. The boards can be made of pharmacists, technicians, and even public members; the main focus is patient safety and setting guidelines for the practice of pharmacy. These boards may require **registration, licensure,** or **certification** to practice as a technician.

Registration – persons are added to a listing but does guarantee the registrants' level of knowledge or expertise

Certification – the person has passed some sort of examination to demonstrate a required level of knowledge

Licensure – the person has met a minimum level of competency that is legally required by the profession

See (Box 1.1) for specific state requirements.

AMERICAN SOCIETY OF HEALTH-SYSTEM PHARMACISTS

In 1942, the **American Society of Health-System Pharmacists (ASHP)** was founded. Its mission is to advocate for pharmacy professionals and support patient medication safety and optimal health. In 1982, the ASHP became the only organization to accredit technician training programs. Throughout the history of the accreditation of training programs, the ASHP has worked

closely with other pharmacy organizations to align duties and responsibilities with training requirements. Standards are written with goals that are required to be achieved by a student attending an ASHP-accredited program based on current practice and collaboration with others in the field, such as the PTCB and the NABP.

The most recent update to the standards occurred in 2018 and supports the advancing role of technicians. There is an entry-level standard that includes basic skills for today's practice settings and an advanced-level standard that includes more patient-related tasks, such as wellness and disease management and supervisory and leadership competencies (these are discussed in Chapter 2).

PHARMACY TECHNICIAN ACCREDITATION COMMISSION

In 2014, the ASHP joined with another organization, the **Accreditation Council for Pharmacy Education (ACPE),** and formed the **Pharmacy Technician Accreditation Commission (PTAC).** This combined group, the ASHP/ACPE, is the accrediting body for technician training programs. The two boards meet separately and vote on a school's program, then grant accreditation if applicable based on a review of the program's curriculum, outcomes, and adherence to standards.

 Tech Note

The ASHP has accredited pharmacy technician training programs since 1982. Some states require graduation from an ASHP/ACPE-accredited program to practice. To find an accredited training program in your state, use the following ASHP link to a directory of all accredited programs: http://accred.ashp.org/aps/pages/directory/technicianProgramDirectory.aspx.

ACCREDITING BUREAU OF HEALTH EDUCATION SCHOOLS

The ABHES offers accreditation for pharmacy technician training programs, and graduates are eligible to sit for the PTCB examination.

NONTRADITIONAL COMPANIES INVOLVED IN PHARMACY

With more than 90% of Americans living within 2 miles of a pharmacy, the push to expand patient care beyond the physician and the pharmacist and participate in wellness and disease prevention has left pharmacies to rely on trained technicians to do the day-to-day tasks and lead pharmacy initiatives.

Companies like Rite Aid, Walgreens, and CVS have dominated the prescription market to date. According to the Centers for Disease Control and Prevention (CDC), about 60% of American adults have at least one chronic illness, such as diabetes or cancer, and more than 40% have more than one chronic illness. This has led to companies like Amazon getting into

Box 1.1

For a list of requirements by state, visit https://nabp.pharmacy/boards-of-pharmacy/.

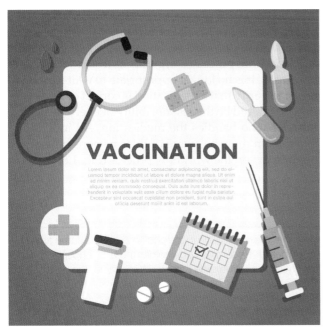

Fig. 1.5 Immunizations are provided at clinics. (Copyright © iStock. com/Guzaliia-Filimonova.)

the healthcare market to share in prescription total expenditures of over $500 billion a year. How do companies that are nonmedical plan to meet the demand for a skilled pharmacy technician workforce to prepare these medications and provide safe medication?

As one example, CVS has created CVS Health, which offers training and internships for several healthcare disciplines, including pharmacy technician (Fig. 1.5). With over 9900 locations and 1100 Minute Clinics, which provide acute care, point-of-care testing such as hepatitis and HIV screenings, and immunizations, the need for skilled and trained medical personnel, including pharmacy technicians, is evident.

> 📮 **Tech Note**
>
> In Idaho, specially trained technicians can give immunizations. They must have CPhT certification and complete a 2-hour self-study and 4-hour live course.

To prepare a trained workforce, Walgreens provides externship sites for many technician training programs and also offers pharmacy education assistance programs to provide financial assistance for individuals going through prepharmacy. In addition to the student benefits of allowing pharmacy technician training programs to use these sites for an externship, the pharmacies can also benefit from the opportunity to work with a potential hire before providing compensation.

Amazon is offering tuition reimbursement and spending up to $700 million to train its workers. Amazon's 2019 acquisition of PillPack, an online pharmacy that ships medications to 49 states, led to a requirement for a pharmacy workforce with advanced training. Nontraditional or nonmedical companies are relying more on education

partnerships to train employees in efficient dispensing and create cost-effective staffing.

A large company's investment in hiring and providing financial assistance to complete a pharmacy technician training program or a specialty training program will create a more invested and highly skilled employee. These workers then become experts in the field, and nonmedical companies depend on this expertise to provide safe medical care in a nontraditional medical environment.

Training a technician to use technology and perform the traditional pharmacist roles with minimum supervision, along with training in leadership skills and specialty training, allows a nonmedical company to compete with traditional pharmacies and maintain a minimal number of highly skilled and highly paid pharmacists alongside a team of advanced pharmacy technicians with significantly lower salaries.

PATIENT SAFETY, ERROR PREVENTION, AND TECHNICIAN TRAINING

Until recently, clerks, assistants, and technicians relied on the pharmacist to check their work and catch any errors. This was because these staff members lacked education and training. But technician roles are expanding, and along with that expansion comes

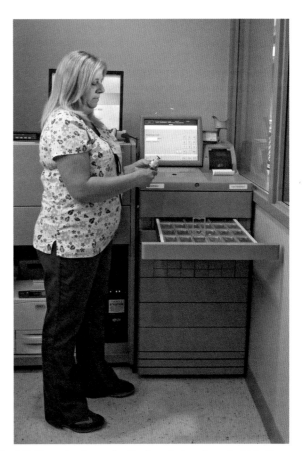

Fig. 1.6 Example of a medication in unit-dose form, individually packaged for dispensing. (From Davis, K., & Guerra, A. [2019]. *Mosby's pharmacy technician* [5th ed.]. St. Louis, MO: Elsevier.)

additional responsibility. Advanced technicians share the common goal of providing the highest-quality care and patient medication safety.

Everyone makes mistakes, but an untrained person handling medication in today's pharmacy environment is unlikely to understand why or how a mistake happened or what to do to prevent a future occurrence. The more training a technician has, the better the technician's understanding of the consequences of errors and just how important it is for the pharmacy to work as a team.

With the expanding roles of technicians in all practice settings, strategies for the prevention of medication errors and an understanding of the impact on the patient and workflow processes are central to the technician's daily tasks. It is no longer appropriate to wait for a pharmacist to verify that a medication is correct or find an error. This should be the responsibility of every healthcare provider who handles the medication. All individuals on the team must be aware of their responsibilities and their impact on the workflow process (Fig. 1.6).

Case Study

You are a CPhT with over 5 years' experience as a technician at a busy hospital pharmacy, and a nurse calls with the following complaint. What would be the appropriate response to this call based on your advanced level of training and experience level?

"Hi, I am Nancy, the RN on duty in Med-Surg today. I just went in the automated dispensing cabinet, and the medication in the pocket was supposed to be Dyazide (hydrochlorothiazide/triamterene), but instead, Maxzide (hydrochlorothiazide/triamterene) was in it. My order is for Dyazide 25 mg daily. Is this the same medication? Can I give this to the patient?"

For untrained technicians, the fact that *hydrochlorothiazide/triamterene* is used in both of the drug names might lead them to conclude that it is acceptable to substitute. As an experienced and certified technician, you should immediately know that the medication in the pocket is not the same as what was ordered. Regardless of whether there is a hospital policy that Dyazide and Maxzide are interchangeable, the medication in the pocket must be changed out because the order is for Dyazide. In addition, if there is a substitution policy in place, the technician should question if both drugs are supposed to be in the cabinet.

Being in an advanced role also would require additional considerations beyond just correcting the problem. The next step is to consider why and how this happened to begin with. Who filled the cabinet? Who checked the final product? Is technology in place, such as barcoding, and if so, was it used? What can be done in the future to prevent this event from happening again? Is there a way to identify the two drugs on the shelf with alert stickers or separate them from each other?

Errors can occur at any time in the process of preparing or dispensing medications. If an error occurs and it is caught before the patient receives the medication, it is still an error. Having advanced training as a technician, participating in the error-prevention process through leadership, and having a high-quality work ethic will result in the most efficient workflow process and the ability to provide the best and safest care for the patient. Being trained in specialty areas or advanced roles creates a team environment, along with the pharmacist and other support personnel, and results in fewer errors.

 Tech Note

The responsibility for errors is part of every technician's job, and a lack of knowledge is not an excuse.

REVIEW QUESTIONS

1. Which of the following organizations provides accredited continuing education for pharmacy professionals?
   a. ASHP
   b. ACPE
   c. PTCE
   d. NABP
2. Which of the following organizations offers the ExCPT certification test?
   a. NHA
   b. PTCB
   c. ASHP
   d. NABP

3. Which of the following organizations grants technician training accreditation?
   a. ASHP
   b. PTAC
   c. NHA
   d. PTCB
4. Everyone is responsible for error prevention EXCEPT:
   a. Certified technician
   b. Front clerk
   c. Pharmacist
   d. All of the above
5. The PTCB began offering a national certification exam in which year?
   a. 1942
   b. 1995

   c. 2014

   d. 2009

6. All of the following are considered common pharmacy technician tasks EXCEPT:

   a. Preparing a patient medical history

   b. Preparing a pediatric suspension

   c. Ordering an out-of-stock medication

   d. Calling an insurance company for more information

7. Which of the following statements is true?

   a. If the state law is stricter than the federal law, the state law must be followed.

   b. If the federal law is stricter than the state law, the state law always overrides the federal law.

   c. The federal law will always be stricter than the state law.

   d. None of the above are true.

8. A technician must register in the state of practice for which reason?

   a. The state BOP requires registration to work in that state.

   b. The federal government requires technicians to register to practice in each state.

   c. The NABP requires all technicians to register with the state to practice.

   d. The ASHP requires technicians to be registered in the state to practice.

9. If a technician is registered, which of the following statements is true?

   a. The technician has been placed on a list and has completed a background check.

   b. The technician has passed a competency-based exam.

   c. The technician has achieved a certain level of competency.

   d. All of the above are true.

10. If a technician is a CPhT, which of the following is true?

   a. The technician has been certified by successfully passing a competency exam.

   b. The technician has met a set of requirements per the state BOP.

   c. The technician has graduated from an accredited program.

   d. The technician is registered with the NABP.

CRITICAL THINKING QUESTIONS

1. As a CPhT, you are preparing a sterile compound and realize that you might have injected the wrong amount of additive drug to a container (a bag). No one saw this, but the pharmacist has already checked the final bag, based on the syringe being drawn back, and the nurse is on the way to pick it up. What should you do?

2. As a Level I technician in your facility, you notice that a new job opening is posted for a more advanced position, a Level II technician trainer. You have been working in the pharmacy for over 2 years and are certified, but you know that in your state, you also need to complete an ASHP-accredited program. Where would you find a listing of the closest accredited program in your area?

REFERENCES

Amazon. *Amazon will pay up to $12,000 for employees to study in these four fields.* https://www.cnbc.com/2018/04/19/amazon-will-pay-up-to-46000-for-employees-to-study-these-4-fields.html.

Amazon. *Amazon to spend $700 million on training employees into the Digital age* https://www.cbsnews.com/news/amazon-to-spend-700-million-training-100000-employees-digital-age/.

CVS Health. https://jobs.cvshealth.com/internships.

National Association of Boards of Pharmacy. www.https://nabp.pharmacy/ https://nabp.pharmacy/wp-content/uploads/2016/07/TF-Technician-Regulations_AM92_Jan1996.pdf.

National Association of Boards of Pharmacy. *Boards of Pharmacy.* https://nabp.pharmacy/boards-of-pharmacy/.

National Association of Boards of Pharmacy. *Evolving Pharmacy Technician Roles Open New Doors, Pose New Regulatory Challenges.* https://nabp.pharmacy/wp-content/uploads/2016/07/Innovations_April_2017_Final.pdf.

NHA. https://www.nhanow.com/docs/default-source/pdfs/exam-documentation/test-plans/nha-2016-excpt-test-plan_public_detail.pdf.

Pharmacy Technician Accreditation Commission (PTAC). https://www.ashp.org/Professional-Development/Technician-Program-Accreditation/ASHP-ACPE-Pharmacy-Technician-Accreditation-Commission.

Pharmacy Technician Certification Board (PTCB). *Career outlook.* https://www.ptcb.org/resources/career-outlook#.XUsnw_ZFzIU.

Pharmacy Technician Certification Board. https://www.ptcb.org/about-ptcb/certification-program-changes.

Pharmacy Times. *Vaccines Administered by Certified Pharmacy Technicians in Idaho.* March 27, 2018. Bergan, Karen. Retrieved August 8, 2019 from https://www.pharmacytimes.com/contributor/karen-berger/2018/03/vaccines-administered-by-certified-pharmacy-technicians-in-idaho.

Training and Skills for Advanced Pharmacy Technician Roles

Learning Objectives

1. Explain the role of the pharmacy in the patient-centered approach.
2. Identify advantages associated with advanced-trained technicians.
3. Discuss costs associated with advanced-trained technicians.
4. Discuss the clinical and operational skills sought by the pharmacy profession in advanced technicians.

Key Terms

American Society of Health-System Pharmacists (ASHP) Organization whose mission is to support pharmacy professionals and promote patient medication safety.

ASHP/ACPE A collaboration between the American Society of Health-System Pharmacists and the Accreditation Council for Pharmacy Education for accrediting technician training courses.

Board of pharmacy (BOP) State agency responsible for licensing, registration, and regulating the responsibilities of pharmacists and technicians.

Certified pharmacy technician (CPhT) A technician who has successfully passed the national certification exam.

Medication reconciliation Process of creating an accurate list of all medications and treatment notes.

National Association of Boards of Pharmacy (NABP) Nonprofit association that protects public health by assisting its member boards of pharmacy and offers programs that promote safe pharmacy practices for the benefit of consumers.

Patient-centered approach A team approach to providing care for patients that includes all parties sharing information and assisting the patient in prevention and ongoing care.

Pharmacists' Patient Care Process (PPCP) Developed by The Joint Commission to collaborate with other healthcare providers to provide patient-centered care.

Pharmacy Technician Certification Board (PTCB) Organization that offers national certification of pharmacy technicians (CPhT).

Point-of-care testing (POCT) As part of the patient-centered approach, early diagnosis and monitoring through tests are used to enhance the patient's overall health.

Point-of-dispensing system (PODS) Temporary area where pharmacy is set up to be the point for medication distribution during disasters.

Strategic National Stockpile (SNS) National supply of medical and life-saving pharmaceuticals and supplies distributed during disasters.

INTRODUCTION

ADVANCING THE ROLES OF PHARMACY

Advanced-trained technicians are becoming more of an integral part of the healthcare team. The job descriptions vary from one practice setting to another, and each state **board of pharmacy (BOP)** has specific guidelines that also vary. With the advancement in high-risk and more dangerous medications, the availability of advanced testing for many diseases, and the focus on better lifestyle choices and the push for prevention, all healthcare providers now have added responsibilities in their professions. The **patient-centered approach** is a basic, three-way approach to treating patients. It includes listening to patients, involving patients in decisions, and informing them of the all aspects of their care. As a pharmacy technician who has received additional training, this role promotes the technician in working directly with patients and being an even more active member of the healthcare team in the information-gathering and communication process (Fig. 2.1).

AN HISTORICAL LOOK AT THE INDUSTRY'S PUSH FOR NATIONAL STANDARDS

Organizations such as the **Pharmacy Technician Certification Board (PTCB)** and **American Society of Health-System Pharmacists (ASHP)** have been working together with state BOPs and the **National Association of Boards of Pharmacy (NABP)** to achieve national standards for technicians for patient safety and the pharmacy's service to the public. A national consensus must include regulations, public sectors, and all aspects of pharmacy practice. This is difficult because each state has the autonomy to decide on regulations and oversight of the pharmacy profession, which must include its interested parties and the public within that state.

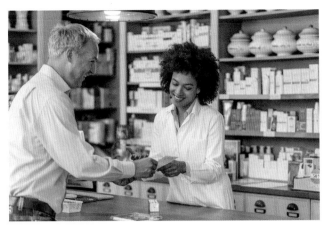

Fig. 2.1 Pharmacy technicians with additional training can work directly with patients. (Copyright © iStock.com/ljubaphoto.)

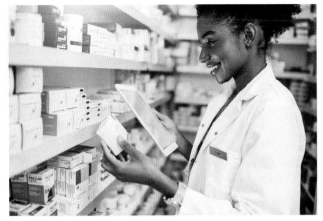

Fig. 2.2 Pharmacy technician performing inventory tasks. (Copyright © iStock.com/Rowan-Jordan.)

Decisions regarding the entry and advanced levels for pharmacy technicians must be evaluated, and different practice settings are also a factor. Technicians in hospital practice, for example, must prepare sterile medications under the guidelines of the US Pharmacopeia (USP), and this requires an advanced knowledge of aseptic technique and an understanding of all critical aspects of microbial transfer possibilities. To address this, the PTCB has added a specialty certification in sterile compounding.

The PTCB has been offering the national certification test since 1995. In 2017, the PTCB sponsored a stakeholder conference that included the ASHP, public stakeholders, and practice representatives to discuss national standards. Key points included the following:

- Agreement for entry-level competency requirements for technicians
- Discussion of variability in state requirements
- Technician accreditation and education requirements
- Technician certification

Speakers such as Christopher Jerry of the Emily Jerry Foundation spoke from the public view of safety and the prevention of medication errors. His daughter, Emily, lost her life as a result of a fatal compounding error made by a pharmacy technician. The need for training to meet the future of pharmacy demands was also discussed. According to the Bureau of Labor Statistics (BLS), there will be a 7% increase in the need for technicians by 2028 (BLS, 2019).

The consensus of the stakeholder meeting identified the need for national standards to provide well-trained pharmacy technicians for patient safety and meeting the needs of the practice.

ADVANTAGES OF ADVANCED-TRAINED TECHNICIANS

As pharmacists' roles becomes more clinical, the day-to-day dispensing and other duties require that there is a well-trained pharmacy staff that can be trusted.

Traditional pharmacy technician tasks are changing every day as this transfer of the pharmacist to a more clinical role is occurring. What once was a pharmacy clerk role has now changed to compounding and value-based medication responsibilities, as discussed in Chapter 4 (Fig. 2.2).

Although the roles are changing for pharmacy technicians, the traditional tasks are still ongoing. Diversifying the staff and creating ladders or positions that enable technicians to work together are essential to efficiency and safety. Some tasks are more complicated and require higher proficiency levels to accomplish, whereas others are less complicated but just as important (Fig. 2.3). With the pharmacy profession moving toward patient-centered care and more clinical roles, the removal of pharmacists from the dispensing process leaves the responsibilities of a well-run pharmacy or department to well-trained technicians. The better trained the technician is, the safer the care is for the patient. With the population of the elderly growing and more of the population having comorbid disease states, we must work together as a unified healthcare profession to meet future patient needs. Each disease affects different body function and organs and having multiple diseases

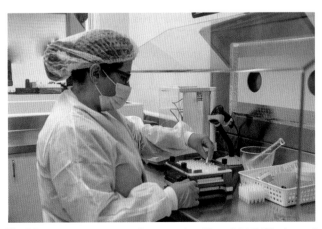

Fig. 2.3 Technician compounding capsules. (Copyright © iStock.com/semyon-lorberg.)

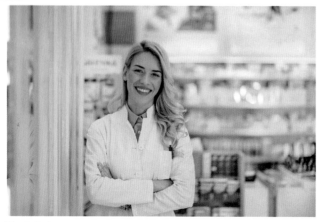

Fig. 2.4 A modern technician. (Copyright © iStock.com/nortonrsx.)

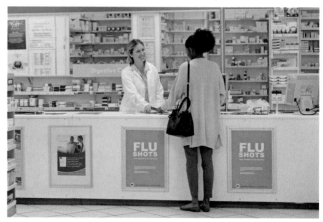

Fig. 2.5 Technician helping a customer who is picking up a prescription. (Copyright © iStock.com/PeopleImages.)

can complicate treatment. For example; treating chronic pain in elderly is difficult because of side effects such as drowsiness or confusion as these may be enhanced due to age and slower metabolism or organ function.

CHARACTERISTICS OF THE MODERN ADVANCED PHARMACY TECHNICIAN

The modern pharmacy includes forward-thinking pharmacy technicians who see their role as a professional and integral part of the pharmacy team. They are competent, energetic, and able to multitask and use critical-thinking skills (Fig. 2.4). They understand the changes in healthcare are focused on a more value-based system with the patient at the center and an overall approach to treatment that includes prevention, awareness, and disease management. These attributes are nurtured through educational programs and advancement opportunities provided by employers. **ASHP/ACPE**, the technician training accrediting body formed through a collaboration between the ASHP and the Accreditation Council for Pharmacy Education (ACPE), offers case studies of advanced technician positions and the associated job descriptions. This is a good resource for opportunities currently in the field; see https://www.ashp.org/Pharmacy-Technician/About-Pharmacy-Technicians/Advanced-Pharmacy-Technician-Roles.

THE COST OF TRAINING THE ADVANCED PHARMACY TECHNICIAN

There is an organizational movement toward companies identifying those technicians who show leadership qualities and who want to take on more responsibilities. Partnerships are emerging between these companies and accredited technician training programs to develop promising employees. Recently, Amazon and Walmart have partnered with Penn Foster Career School to provide pharmacy technician training education. This is costly for companies because they often reimburse the employee or pay for national certification tests at a minimum. The upside is that pharmacists can rely on well-trained technicians to perform at a higher level of quality, which allows them to spend more time on patient care.

Healthcare is more of a value-based decision today, as patients shop around for insurance, providers, and pharmacies based on cost, along with other factors. That means pharmacies that hire technicians must consider their training and ability to perform advanced roles. An organization with all entry-level technicians may not have the ability to manage the number of prescriptions processed compared with one that has several advanced technicians who are trusted with more complicated tasks or leadership roles. Customer service and public perception of an organization can make or break pharmacies in this competitive healthcare environment (Fig. 2.5). The average person picking up a prescription demands attention from the pharmacist for questions and counseling, and without a trusted pool of trained technicians to do the regular, everyday dispensing, they would not have the time. The pharmacist must have confidence in the technicians' ability, or the organization will not have the ability to address each patient's individual needs.

Today's insurance offerings support a value-based approach, including incentives for lifestyle changes to better manage existing disease states (Fig. 2.6). In this value-based medication environment, patients are offered lower copays, spending accounts, and other incentives to promote wellness and better management of their health. Participating providers,

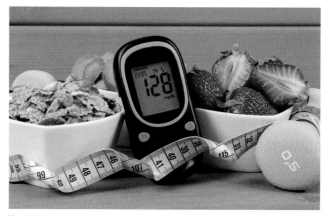

Fig. 2.6 Diabetes management. (Copyright © iStock.com/ratmaner.)

including pharmacies, must compete and provide the most efficient services while reducing operating costs, in some cases with fewer staff members. If patients are not satisfied with the professional services offered, they will choose another provider to find the level of care they are paying for. For pharmacies, this means having a well-trained staff and thinking outside the box. distributing the workload and responsibilities to advanced-trained technicians provides for better-quality services for the patient. As part of providing quality services, the public perception of a pharmacy and the staff is critical. Most of the public sees technicians as trained professionals who work alongside the pharmacist, and many do not realize that, in some instances, they are not required to complete training or advanced degrees to qualify for employment (Fig. 2.7). This has forced some facilities to create internal training programs to promote technicians to advanced positions with additional responsibilities. Interactions with patients are an integral part of the overall process of patient-centered care, and the confidence level a patient has for an advanced-trained technician improves medication compliance and provides a more efficient system. Many are establishing in-house training programs and creating levels of technicians in order to cut cost without compromising the care offered to the patient.

Even though training takes time from a facility's daily routine and workflow, the benefits outweigh the cost because it creates a more competent professionals who interact as one team. Clinically oriented pharmacy technicians can provide support and expertise by taking over some of the pharmacist's clerical, data-collection, and project-management responsibilities. This can include screening disease outcomes or conditions, monitoring lab results, or tracking medication errors and reporting opportunities. The time that it takes for these tasks to be completed by an advanced-trained technician allows pharmacists to perform their clinical role and streamline clinical and operational services. The expansion of services through clinical technicians allows a facility to use more technician positions while decreasing the number of higher-paid pharmacists.

CLINICAL AND OPERATIONAL SKILLS FOR ADVANCED TECHNICIAN ROLES

For a certified technician, a common way to progress to advanced roles is to work in several traditional pharmacy technician roles and show initiative and good communication skills. Having basic computer skills, the ability to work independently, and the ability to make confident decisions are qualities that employers look for when choosing candidates for advanced roles.

CLINICAL SKILLS OF THE ADVANCED TECHNICIAN

Direct interaction with the other healthcare staff and the ability to communicate across disciplines are responsibilities and qualities expected of advanced technicians. Performing clinical roles, such as **point-of-care testing (POCT)**, and participating in the **Pharmacist's Patient Care Process (PPCP)** require a basic pharmacology understanding and the ability to support the pharmacist in the collection, observation, and recording of information (Fig. 2.8).

The PPCP is a new process that was introduced by The Joint Commission and as part of the Patient Protection and Affordable Care Act. As part of this act, Medicare must provide coverage for wellness and preventive services. This process requires working directly with patients and other healthcare team members, including third-party providers, to record demographic and condition or disease information. In addition, there is a collaborative wellness and disease prevention plan designed for each patient to optimize health and medication adherence. The PPCP also addresses ways to manage the diseases or other predisposed diseases that patients face. Comorbid diseases, such as diabetes and high blood pressure, affect the patient's overall health, and lifestyle changes can greatly

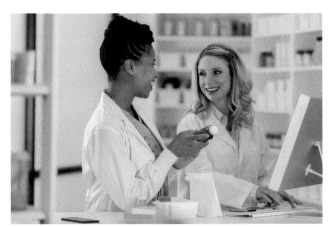

Fig. 2.7 Collaboration between the technician and the pharmacist. (Copyright © iStock.com/SDI-Productions.)

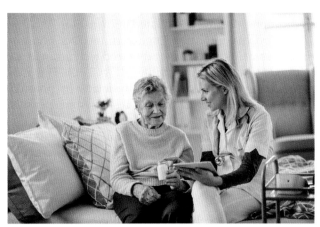

Fig. 2.8 Technician interviewing a patient. (Copyright © iStock.com/ Halfpoint.)

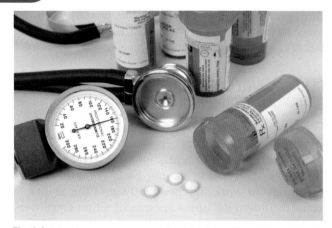

Fig. 2.9 Blood pressure meter and medications. (Copyright © iStock.com/doublediamondphoto.)

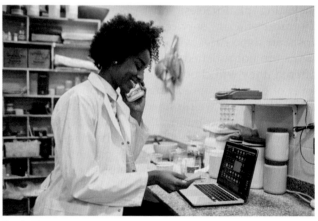

Fig. 2.10 Technician verifying a patient's history with the physician's office. (Copyright © iStock.com/alvarez.)

increase quality of life (Fig. 2.9). Advanced technicians can support and work along with the pharmacist to assist in many support roles in the PPCP process, such as the following:

- Anticoagulation or blood draws
- Immunizations
- Compliance and patient safety
- **Medication reconciliation**
- Preadmission histories
- Education regarding smoking, alcohol, diet, and exercise

Many third-party insurance providers require employees to maintain a point-value system that monitors lifestyle and preventive testing or screening as part of a wellness-promotion approach. As part of this approach, advanced pharmacy technicians can be trained to perform POCT, such as cholesterol screening and glucose testing, and education related to diet, smoking and alcohol use cessation, and exercise.

Taking medication histories requires advanced clinical skills to interpret and record disease processes and test and lab values, as well as an overall understanding of pharmacology and medical terminology. Completing medication reconciliation or medication therapy management documentation for a patient's medical records includes correct spelling of diseases, medications, dosing, and related information. As a part of this process, indicators predetermined for pharmacist assessments require the advanced technician to use competent investigative abilities (Fig. 2.10). This may require communication with physicians or pharmacists to determine refill patterns, results from specialist appointments or tests, and medication compliance.

The advanced technician clinical skills in today's modern pharmacy include direct patient instruction regarding side effects, medication adherence, The advanced technician can also perform simple POCT. This can include immunizations; A1C tests; and screenings for hepatitis C, fecal blood, and other similar tests. Many chain and large drugstores house ambulatory or wellness-type clinics. The staffing may include

medical assistants, physician's assistants, nurses, and advanced technicians. Patients can use these services as referrals for testing, wellness, or disease-prevention consultations with the pharmacist, or immunizations, rather than the traditional physician's office visit (Fig. 2.11).

Good communication is also key to the advanced technician's clinical skills. Often, patients will have discrepancies with medications, such as dosing or multiple physician prescriptions for similar medications (Fig. 2.12). Patients may not understand that they are taking two medications that are just the brand and generic versions of the same drug or that a dose was decreased or stopped. Clarifying or reconciling the records requires advanced technicians to understand the issue and work directly with another healthcare provider to get clear answers and a solution. They must use computer skills to review prescription histories, have an understanding of multiple third-party plans and formularies, and be able to communicate with the different parties for resolution.

Performing in emergencies or in a disaster role requires advanced technician skills in cardiopulmonary

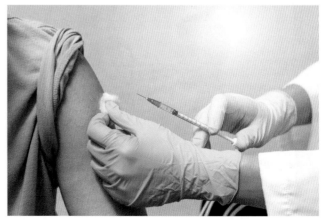

Fig. 2.11 Patient getting a flu vaccine. (Copyright © iStock.com/Pornpak_Khunatorn.)

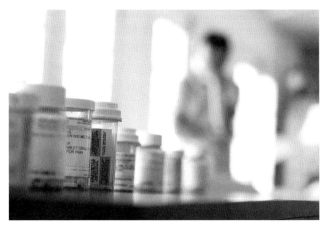

Fig. 2.12 Multiple prescription bottles. (Copyright © iStock.com/DNY59.)

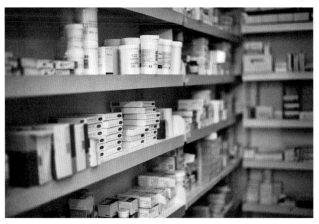

Fig. 2.14 Medications stored on shelves for the Strategic National Stockpile (SNS). (Copyright © iStock.com/Tinpixels.)

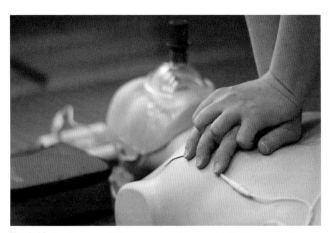

Fig. 2.13 Performing CPR in training. (Copyright © iStock.com/DarrenTownsend.)

resuscitation (CPR) and other related skills (Fig. 2.13). The advanced technician may be required to assist with life-threatening situations anywhere and at any time. First-aid certification is also a clinical skill that the advanced technician should maintain. Participating in a code situation and using a crash cart, for instance, may require an advanced understanding of the types of medications and the dosing and administration of medications maintained in the cart, as well as the inventory process for replacement and stocking. With today's current environment, each state has disaster plans for weather-related events, natural disasters, and terrorist events. It's all hands on deck in such cases, but advanced technicians can often work

in leadership roles for temporary **point-of-dispensing systems (PODSs)** or stations manned during an event. This frees up pharmacists to work in a more clinical role when there may be a shortage of physicians. In disasters, it is important to maintain records and know the state's policy for each type of event. Records must be kept, and this often requires handwritten documentation because of loss of power or internet capabilities during disaster situations.

In addition to participation during a disaster event, preparation for such events is also critical. Advanced technicians should have a clinical understanding of the types of medications and supplies proved by the **Strategic National Stockpile (SNS)**. This is a stockpile of emergency medications and supplies maintained by hospitals, pharmacies, and other public facilities such as the public health department. Typical medications include antibiotics, immunizations, and emergency drugs. The advanced technician must maintain in-date stock and have an understanding of the classes of medications and the uses for each one maintained in inventory (Fig. 2.14).

OPERATIONAL SKILLS OF THE ADVANCED TECHNICIAN

Today's advanced technician performs more complicated operational tasks than before. The day-to-day activities of dispensing, inventory management, workflow, and scheduling are just some of these tasks.

Pharmacy and technician mangers look to advanced technicians to know the inventory needs of the pharmacy better than themselves. They understand the cycling and financial costs of medications because they are directly involved in these processes. They are often in positions of leadership for inventory management and maintain efficient stocking levels. They interact directly with the Pharmacy and Therapeutics (P&T) Committee and other healthcare providers to maintain formularies. The P&T group includes nurses, pharmacists, physicians, and other healthcare providers and

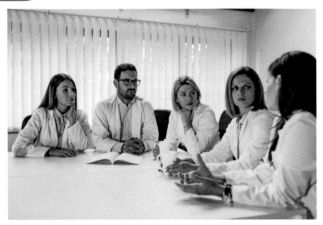

Fig. 2.15 Pharmacy and Therapeutics (P&T) Committee meeting in a hospital. (Copyright © iStock.com/nortonrsx.)

determines lists of approved medications to help align physicians' needs with cost-effective medication therapy for the patient and facility (Fig. 2.15).

Advanced technicians must have skills in workflow and efficient management of departments. This involves task assignments, scheduling of staff, and training of new technicians. A well-trained advanced technician understands the strengths and weaknesses of the technician staff and what is required to be efficient in dispensing and providing quality care. This requires an understanding of time management, communication, leadership, and multitasking. Advanced technicians must have the ability to manage different personalities and conflicts within a department while keeping the day-to-day operations running smoothly.

Proficiency with technology is another skill required for the advanced roles of technicians (Fig. 2.16). Today's pharmacy is driven by some of the most efficient distribution and tracking systems available. In some states, the "tech check tech" (TCT) system is used. This is the process of an advanced technician checking another technician's accuracy in the order-filling process. This is usually limited to the filling of automated dispensing machines or unit-dose batches of refills in institutional settings. Knowledge of the technology being used and medication information, such as brand and generic versions of drugs, is required to be accurate in this process. Other technology managed by advanced technicians includes the automation used in sterile compounding, robotic filling machines, and repacking systems from bulk to unit dose (Fig. 2.17).

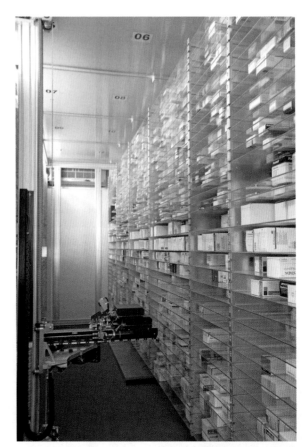

Fig. 2.16 A computer-automated pharmacy stockroom. (Copyright © iStock.com/clu.)

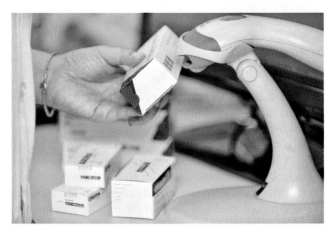

Fig. 2.17 Using barcoding technology for verification of correct medications. (Copyright © iStock.com/MJ_Prototype.)

Evaluating pharmacy operations and participating in a department's quality control efforts are part of the modern advanced technician's roles. This requires knowledge in current regulations for state and national organizational standards, an understanding of facility policies, and critical-thinking skills. In an effort to evaluate potential harmful medications, therapy duplications or adverse interactions can be the "first stop" for an advanced technician reviewing a department process or patient record. Having a good understanding of how to filter or discern information and

---

💬 **Tech Note**

There are 17 states (California, Colorado, Idaho, Iowa, Kansas, Kentucky, Illinois, Michigan, Minnesota, Montana, North Dakota, North Carolina, Maryland, South Carolina, Ohio, Oregon, and Washington) that allow pharmacy technicians to check the work of other technicians in hospital and institutional or community settings through the TCT (Tech Check Tech) program (National Association of Boards of Pharmacy [NABP], 2009)

the ability to use a set of operational resources to create a potential plan for correction are advanced skills that allow the technician to be an extremely valuable team member.

Advanced technicians are the experts on insurance and third-party reimbursement in today's pharmacy. Because they are involved in the day-to-day activities and see almost every prescription in some part of the dispensing process, they are most current with the plans and requirements for billing. Pharmacy mangers look to them for feedback on what is working and what would be the best ways to improve efficiency and patient care while cutting costs. Today's competitive market requires a constant evaluation to ensure the facility is providing quality patient-centered care and services while reducing waste and using every resource to the fullest.

The need for advanced technicians will only increase with the advancements in technology, a number of patients living longer, and the advances in medication and disease management. The pharmacist's roles are becoming more and more clinical in nature, and the day-to-day activities of the pharmacy are being left to well-trained staff who are often managed by experienced advanced technicians. Many facilities are being forced to streamline services because of reimbursements and budget restraints, so future leadership is looking to maximize services by employing fewer, more highly trained staff. Advanced technicians who choose to pursue and meet the challenging operational and clinical skills needed today are experiencing better compensation and respect and are making a significant contribution to the profession.

Case Study

You are a **certified pharmacy technician (CPhT)** with over 5 years' experience as a technician at a busy community pharmacy, and you notice a position posting for a new clinic opening within the pharmacy. It is for a "technician manager." Describe at least two operational and two clinical skills that are needed to be the best possible candidate.

Operational skills would include the ability to organize activities and prepare a staffing schedule, inventory management experience, experience with technology and good computer skills, multitasking abilities, and insurance/billing knowledge.

Clinical skills would include the ability to perform POCT, the ability to review patient profiles and complete history documentation, good communications skills, a good understanding of pharmacology, and knowledge of medical terms.

REVIEW QUESTIONS

1. Which of the following involves recording a patient's history and determining a plan for wellness and disease management?
   a. POCT
   b. PPCP
   c. PTCB
   d. NABP
2. All of the following states allow TCT EXCEPT:
   a. North Dakota
   b. South Carolina
   c. Texas
   d. California
3. Which group determines a medication formulary within an organization?
   a. ASHP
   b. P&T
   c. NABP
   d. PTCB
4. Which type of insurance programs offers patients incentives for taking better care of themselves?
   a. POD
   b. Value based
   c. Point of care
   d. Patient-centered care
5. The patient-centered approach to treating patients includes which of the following?
   a. Interviewing the patient
   b. Involving the patient in decisions
   c. Informing the patient of all options
   d. All of the above
6. All of the following are common types of POCT EXCEPT:
   a. P&T
   b. Fecal blood
   c. A1C
   d. Hepatitis C
7. Which of the following statements is true regarding PPCP?
   a. Can include education on smoking cessation
   b. Can include history of current medications
   c. Can include diabetes testing and monitoring
   d. All of the above
8. Which of the following are often considered by employers to determine candidates for advanced technician opportunities?
   a. Good computer skills
   b. Ability to work independently
   c. Good decision-making skills
   d. All of the above

9. The main technician tasks used to assist the pharmacist in the PPCP include all of the following EXCEPT:
   a. Observation
   b. Collection
   c. Documentation
   d. Counseling

10. An advanced technician who checks another technician's accuracy when filling a medication would be considered part of which process?
    a. TCT
    b. POCT
    c. PPCP
    d. Patient-centered care

CRITICAL THINKING QUESTIONS

1. You are interviewing a patient and creating a history of medications. The patient notes that the prescription is obtained from two pharmacies. What would you do first in order to obtain the most accurate record?

2. You have been working as a technician for over 5 years, and you want to see what type of advanced roles are out there. Where would you find a resource describing the different positions available?

REFERENCES

ASHP. *Advanced Technician Roles: Case Studies.* Retrieved https://www.ashp.org/Pharmacy-Technician/About-Pharmacy-Technicians/Advanced-Pharmacy-Technician-Roles.

Barker, Alex. (June 2015). *9 Ways Pharmacy Technician roles are Changing.* https://www.pharmacytimes.com/contributor/alex-barker-pharmd/2015/06/9-new-ways-pharmacy-technician-roles-are-changing.

Bureau of Labor and Statistics (BLS). Retrieved August 26, 2019 from https://www.bls.gov/ooh/healthcare/pharmacy-technicians.htm.

Kreckel, Peter. (2018, May 7). *It's Time to Rethink Pharmacy Tech Staffing.* https://www.drugtopics.com/viewpoints/its-time-rethink-pharmacy-tech-staffing.

Krizner, Ken. (Jun 5, 2019). *Training Techs for more responsibility.* https://www.drugtopics.com/training/training-technicians-more-responsibility.

Medscape. Tech-Check-Tech. 2011. Retrieved September 26. 2019 from https://www.medscape.com/viewarticle/750654_5.

Zellmer, William A., McAllister, Everett B., Silvester, Janet A., & Vlasses, Peter H. (September 1, 2017). Toward uniform standards for pharmacy technicians: Summary of the 2017 Pharmacy Technician Stakeholder Consensus Conference. *American Journal of Health-System Pharmacy, 74*(17), 1321–1332. https://doi.org/10.2146/ajhp170283.

Leadership and Management Skills

Learning Objectives

1. Discuss leadership skills that can expand opportunities for advanced technician roles.
2. Discuss management skills for advanced technicians.
3. Explain how good leadership and management skills can enable a healthcare team to be more effective.
4. Describe ways advanced technicians in leadership roles can enhance patient safety and efficiency in providing medication services.

Key Terms

Career ladder System using experience and knowledge to determine levels of responsibilities.

Patient-centered care A team approach to providing care for patients that includes all parties sharing information and assisting the patient in prevention and ongoing care.

Tiers Levels of responsibilities.

INTRODUCTION

A SNAPSHOT OF THE ADVANCED TECHNICIAN IN LEADERSHIP ROLES

Advanced-trained technicians must not only possess skills and knowledge to perform tasks associated with higher-level medication processes, but they must also be leaders (Fig. 3.1). This requires experience, good judgment, and confidence in their ability to perform the medication-related tasks required while acting in the role of a leader. Showing these leadership and management qualities also gains pharmacists' trust, which gives them more time to perform their clinical role. Being a leader inspires others to do their best and meet challenges that push them out of their comfort area. This is the way an advanced technician in a management role can mentor and encourage less experienced technicians to be able to move up the ladder to advanced or specialty positions. Every person on the team has an important role, and a collaborative team increases efficiency and improves patient safety.

Today's pharmacy often uses **tiers** or **career ladders** for the technicians. The advanced technician roles in this scenario require some leadership or management roles and specialty roles. Having experience in the field and the skills to interact and communicate well with each team member and patients is critical to the advanced technician in any role (Fig. 3.2).

ADVANCED TECHNICIAN LEADER ROLES

An advanced technician should encourage and inspire others to do their best. Directing others to share and work toward a common mission is a challenge and requires an understanding of the team's members as individuals. Working with their strengths and weaknesses and guiding them by example will likely motivate them to do their best. Within today's pharmacy structure, there is a complex set of services that now includes more focus on the **patient-centered care** approach. This complicates the process for day-to-day activities and requires advanced technicians to specialize in areas to meet the increasing patient expectations. Motivating and mentoring technicians in a "tier" environment encourages technicians at all levels to perform at their highest best and maximizes efficiency for the department.

 Tech Note

A good leader knows how important it is to use every information source available. It is not as important to know all the answers but to know *where* to find them (Fig. 3.3).

LEADERSHIP SKILLS OF ADVANCED TECHNICIANS

Leadership also includes integrity. If advanced technicians are not honest and trustworthy, how could they ever expect someone to follow their lead? Being in

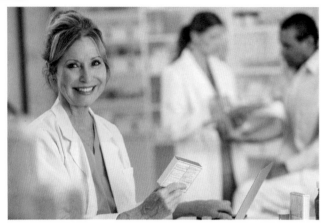

Fig. 3.1 Pharmacy team members working together for the patient. (Copyright © iStock.com/SDI-Productions.)

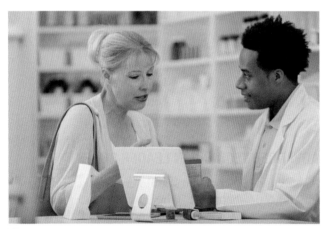

Fig. 3.2 Technician communicating with a senior patient. (Copyright © iStock.com/SDI-Productions.)

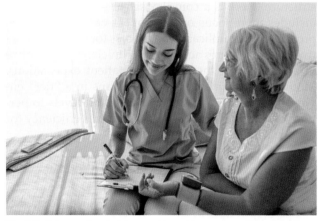

Fig. 3.3 Advanced technician working with a patient. (Copyright © iStock.com/dragana991.)

direct contact with patients and working side by side with the healthcare team must include ethical behavior.

Good leaders also have confidence in themselves and in those they lead. Having experience in the field and demonstrating the ability to collaborate within and outside the department help minimize medication errors. Interacting with the other technicians and support staff with a confident attitude when performing each task allows for a positive work environment and a much more productive and wiser use of resources.

Being a good communicator is also a key aspect of the leadership roles of advanced technicians. Being able to share a vision or a common goal and motivate technicians to work together will create a safe and productive atmosphere for the patient. Providing services in today's pharmacy includes direct interaction between the advanced technician and the patient. This may be a "meds to beds" approach, in which the technician may collect medication histories or answer nonclinical questions, such as questions regarding storage or expiration dates. The ability to communicate well with colleagues and other professionals whose main goal is to take care of the patient enables a leader to share useful information correctly.

Being able to make decisions is another key leadership quality for the advanced technician in a management position. Knowing when to consult key people and understanding the consequences of a decision are essential. As a leader, the advanced technician may be asked to make certain day-to-day decisions that affect more than just the department. For example, a decision may be one that affects the entire organization and requires additional information. Knowing when to ask questions and thinking through all the elements of the decision are the signs of a good leader.

Knowing that you cannot do everything and being able to delegate are also key leadership qualities. If a task is assigned, provide the person with the resources to be successful in its completion. A good leader will have the ability to identify and trust someone to complete the job. In addition, the delegate now has the ability to take ownership in the process or work, and this allows them to grow.

Being accountable is another important attribute. Being committed to a goal, working through obstacles, and holding subordinates accountable will ensure the problem is solved or the task is completed. This may require "thinking outside the box" or finding a nontraditional approach to the problem.

> **Tech Note**
>
> Just because the department may be experiencing a staff shortage or limited resources does not mean the patient shouldn't get the best care available.

In today's pharmacy, one of the most important leadership qualities is creativity or innovation. The reimbursement and staffing decreases have left many pharmacies to do more with less to stay competitive. This is a great place for the advanced technician to shine. With an understanding of workflow, inventory, staffing, and how to delegate responsibilities appropriately, the advanced technician is indispensable.

ADVANCED TECHNICIAN AS MANAGERS

Advanced technicians can perform in management roles and bring expertise and knowledge in many ways. This may be managing specialty areas, performing as coordinators, or acting as evaluators or trainers. In today's pharmacy, technicians who have experience and show leadership qualities are also serving as intermediate supervisors and first-level managers. They may lead a team of other technicians or provide high-level support in specialty areas. Management of a busy pharmacy requires a collaborative team approach to ensure the overall organization is functioning properly. Advanced technicians can contribute to this by demonstrating management skills that propel the mission of the department and facilitate an easy flow of activity.

MANAGEMENT SKILLS OF THE ADVANCED TECHNICIAN

One of the most important management skills is the demonstration of technical skills. Advanced technicians should have experience in the field and show that they can perform tasks with little supervision. They must understand different types of technology and how to use each to achieve the goals set by the organization. This is important because the top leadership trusts that the tasks under the supervision of the advanced technician will be completed correctly and with very minimal supervision. Advanced technicians are an integral part of the workflow process, and if they do not understand the technical tasks required in their position and those of other team members, it can cause subsequent processes to be affected (Fig. 3.4).

Another key skill is imagination or conceptual skills. These are skills that involve analyzing a problem, formulating processes, and determining an appropriate outcome. Often in the advanced role, there may be tasks assigned to the technician that are presented as just a broad concept or idea. This requires the ability to break a project into manageable steps and use resources to get the outcome needed. The high-level supervisor wants advanced technicians to take on the assignment and use their expertise and the resources provided to complete the necessary tasks. Advanced technicians must start with the basic concept, analyze and diagnose the best options, and determine responsible parties. They will use their knowledge of the organization's overall mission, technical skills, and understanding of the staff they supervise to complete the task. This process of delegation allows an intermediate manager to work through an issue and provide the high-level supervisor with a solution that can then be implemented into the overall process.

Delegation is an important attribute of the advanced technician serving in a management role. Knowing the staff and matching the right assignment based on skills and the ability for completion are necessary to keep the department on task and running smoothly. Having experience in the field allows for a better understanding of what it takes to complete the assignment, and when delegation is done properly, the results can be quick and produce optimal results.

> **Tech Note**
>
> A good manager allows others to perform a task assigned without micromanaging, which can allow the person to grow and become a future leader.

The advanced technician manager must be able to plan and problem solve. Once an assignment is presented, it must stay within the limits of available resources and align with the mission of the department or organization. For intermediate supervisors, this will require strategies and identifying achievable goals for subordinates. It isn't just about planning to get a task done but also integration and remaining within limits of budget and labor because the outcome will affect others within the department as well as outside. The technicians look to the manager to formulate a plan and determine each of their roles in it. Ultimately, the manager's supervisor will expect results from the manager.

One of the most important management skills that the advanced technician should have is decision-making abilities. High-level managers answer to many different people and depend on the lower management positions to work toward a common goal and get the job done. Making a poor decision not only affects a manager's immediate area but also the overall organization. Relying on past experiences as a technician and communicating and working in conjunction with others on the team to make a good decision will prevent conflict and facilitate the best outcome (Fig. 3.5).

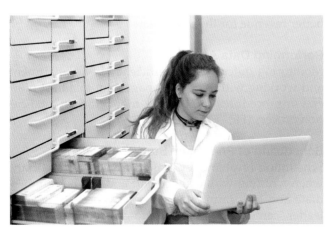

Fig. 3.4 Advanced technician working with a complex inventory system. (Copyright © iStock.com/Maica.)

Case Study

You are a Level III technician in a busy hospital and have four technicians under your supervision. Your area of focus is management of the automated dispensing cabinet (ADC) area. This includes all aspects of inventory control, management of the four technicians, and working directly with the nursing staff on the floor.

The supervising pharmacist comes to you to report that a nurse on the critical care unit (CCU) states that she is constantly out of drugs in her cabinet and has asked a couple of technicians a few times to increase the periodic automatic replenishment (PAR) level if possible. This is the minimum quantity of an item that must be kept on hand. You remember a conversation a week ago regarding this, and you asked one of your technicians to check on this and put in a request to change the PAR. Following this conversation with your supervisor, you talk to the technician

regarding this task assignment. She states she missed the training from you on this process because she was out sick, and you had told her you would reschedule. She asked another technician to do this and never heard if that technician did or not. You realize you never rescheduled the training.

Could this have been avoided? What would you do to correct this issue?

Being in a management role requires good planning and delegation skills. This situation could have been avoided by rescheduling the training and reassigning the task that day. In the management role, you must understand the responsibilities of your position and how they can ultimately affect the patient. Higher management sees this as part of your job, and it is essential in gaining their trust and securing their confidence.

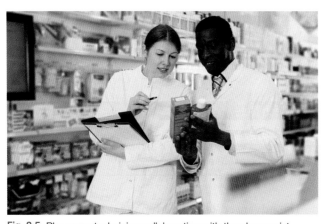

Fig. 3.5 Pharmacy technician collaborating with the pharmacist regarding stocking a medication. (Copyright © iStock.com/JackF.)

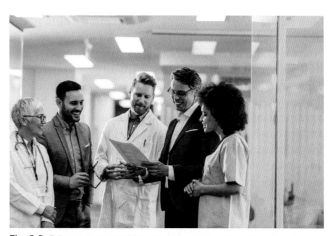

Fig. 3.6 Primary care providers and pharmacy personnel discussing patient outcomes. (Copyright © iStock.com/skynesher.)

COMMON MANAGEMENT DUTIES PERFORMED BY THE ADVANCED TECHNICIAN LEADER OR MANAGER

The advanced technician in a leadership or management position can play a significant role in many areas. There are many opportunities in today's pharmacy structure, all of which include the use of the advanced technician's skills, experience, and leadership qualities, as described in the following subsections.

Serving on Committees

Serving on committees allows the constant flow of information and facilitates a collaborative approach to patient care. In a leadership role, the advanced technician can share best practices and relay information to others on the team to work toward a common patient-centered goal. These could be medication safety, quality assurance, analytics, or formulary-related committees (Fig. 3.6).

Resolving Billing Issues and Inventory Management

Reimbursement is often time based. Over a certain amount of time, reimbursement is prorated. Knowing how to bill properly and in a timely manner allows for better revenue for the pharmacy.

Performing Data Analysis

Monitoring outcomes and efficiency in a department and working with higher management to adjust policies or procedures can create a more efficient medication process (Fig. 3.7).

Scheduling of Pharmacy Staff/Technicians

Scheduling of pharmacy staff is especially important when working with a short staff and has both immediate and long-term effects. The advanced technician leader can ensure that day-to-day operations run smoothly and that work is done in a timely manner through proper scheduling.

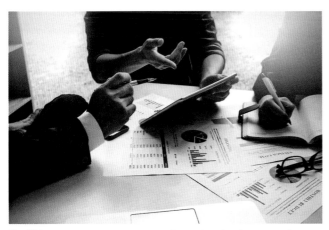

Fig. 3.7 Pharmacy team members discussing the department's monthly costs. (Copyright © iStock.com/Jirapong-Manustrong.)

Answering Questions and Training Technicians

Assisting technicians or staff at a lower level (tier) is important while acting in an interim supervisory position. The use of experience and past knowledge is key to creating a team environment and being efficient.

Being a Liaison With Other Departments

Communicating best practices or discussing issues that affect the way the system performs as a complete healthcare team is important for the delivery of patient-centered care. The advanced technician leader or manager can bridge the gap between the requirements of day-to-day activities and the overall mission of the department (Fig. 3.8).

Performing Evaluations and Monitoring the Performance of Technicians

The performance of technicians is often best evaluated by someone who is with the employees daily. Pharmacist managers rely on the advanced technician to train and supervise employees and use a reporting structure for improvement plans or changes as needed.

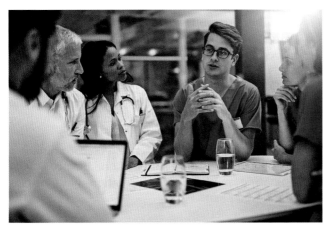

Fig. 3.8 Hospital meeting with different departments, including an analyst technician. (Copyright © iStock.com/Cecilie_Arcurs.)

ADVANCED TECHNICIANS' CONTRIBUTION TO TEAM EFFICIENCY

Serving as a leader or manager in the pharmacy can increase the overall team or department's efficiency. With reimbursement cuts and staffing at a minimum as cost reductions continue, pharmacies must use their resources more efficiently, and this includes placing advanced technicians in intermediate or higher leadership positions.

The push to reinforce patient participation and increase satisfaction with services around individual health and wellness benefits is key to the future of healthcare. This requires pharmacists to serve in a more clinical role, which leaves the day-to-day activities to a trusted staff in a well-run department. Expanding the responsibilities of the advanced technician allows more of them to have more direct interaction with patients. This provides the pharmacy with the ability to offer additional services, such as immunizations, point-of-care testing, and the collection of medication histories. Advanced technicians can greatly participate in the reduction of errors. With the ratio of 3 technicians to every one pharmacist in most states averaging, this creates a scenario of several technicians in a department who can be divided into tiers or career ladders, allowing a smaller staff of pharmacists to have additional time to collaborate with the primary caregivers and the patient.

ADVANCED TECHNICIAN EFFECT ON PATIENT SAFETY AND REDUCTION OF MEDICATION ERRORS

The use of advanced technicians in leadership roles fosters an atmosphere of collaboration inside and outside the organization. Sharing a common goal of patient-centered care allows the technician to interact with nursing and other caregivers on an intermediate supervisory level. This collaboration can help reduce errors and improve patient safety. Advanced technicians can assist in reducing medication errors in many ways. Reviewing a patient's medication history can catch adherence issues, flag untimely fills or refills, and prevent future medication errors or even death in some cases. Using the information gathered and sharing recommendations with others can decrease patient harm and provide background information. This will expand the pharmacist's available consulting time.

 Tech Note

Over 7000 deaths occur from medication errors each year (Kohn et al., 2000).

Healthcare systems today have a vast array of numerous departments and complex services. Good communication among all the different services and caregivers is essential to provide the safest and most

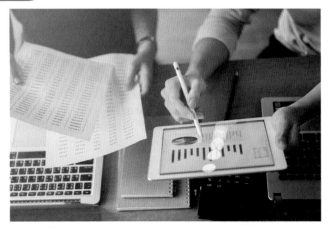

Fig. 3.9 Staff from the hospital and pharmacy discussing the organization's new business concept. (Copyright © iStock.com/Chainarong-Prasertthai.)

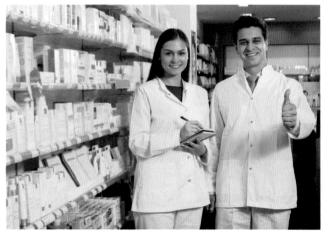

Fig. 3.10 Pharmacist and advanced technician demonstrating teamwork. (Copyright © iStock.com/JackF.)

efficient care for the patient. However, this also sets the stage for one area to not know what the others are doing, which can lead to medication errors and duplication of services. When advanced technicians have leadership roles, they are able to use their higher level of cognitive ability and experience to analyze processes and create better outcomes. They are able to make decisions that will allow the department to provide the patient with the best-quality services available.

Many pharmacies use advanced technicians in quality assurance and control programs. In this role, advanced technicians gather data, assist in policy changes, run and review reports, and help design the organizational plan for services. By serving in intermediate supervisory positions, they can provide a perspective on how basic day-to-day activities fit within the overall mission of the department (Fig. 3.9).

LEADERSHIP AND MANAGEMENT OPPORTUNITIES FOR ADVANCED TECHNICIANS IN THE FUTURE

Pharmacy practice is changing daily. The goals of healthcare and providing quality services with fewer resources are required for pharmacies to stay competitive today. The use of experienced advanced technicians in intermediate supervisory positions provides a valuable resource for an organization to provide the best care for the patient.

Good leaders don't just see today. They see the future as rewarding, and in some cases, being an advanced technician in a leadership position is a step toward the next level of pharmacist. Numerous pharmacies offer tiers or levels so that the technician can advance through a career ladder. The rewards of advancement most often include increased salary, the ability to coach and mentor others, and the respect and satisfaction of being recognized in an advanced technician leadership role (Fig. 3.10).

REVIEW QUESTIONS

1. Which of the following is a leadership skill that demonstrates the ability to cover the shift of a technician who is unable to work?
   a. Delegation
   b. Communication
   c. Experience in field
   d. Integrity
2. Which term best describes the process of advancing through mastery of different levels of responsibilities?
   a. Experience
   b. Career ladder
   c. Delegation
   d. Integrity
3. Which term is used to describe sharing information about the overall care and wellness of the patient?
   a. Patient-focused care
   b. Patient-centered care
   c. Point-of-care testing
   d. Patient care process
4. All of the following describe changes in the pharmacy setting commonly seen today EXCEPT:
   a. Increase of staff to meet patient needs
   b. Higher reimbursement for more expensive treatments
   c. Decrease in staffing
   d. Use of intermediate advanced technician positions
5. The role of advanced technicians in the patient-centered care approach includes which of the following?
   a. Collaboration through serving on committees
   b. Collecting a patient's medication history
   c. Sharing medication information with nurses and other staff
   d. All of the above

6. All of the following are common results from working in an advanced technician leadership role EXCEPT:
   a. Respect
   b. Increased salary
   c. Job satisfaction
   d. Decreased responsibility
7. What is the current average ratio of technicians to pharmacists in the country?
   a. 2:1
   b. 3:1
   c. 4:1
   d. 6:1
8. Leadership skills that are often used by employers to determine candidates for advanced technician opportunities include which of the following?
   a. Good communication skills
   b. Ability to interact with others
   c. Good decision-making skills
   d. All of the above
9. A snapshot of the advanced technician's leadership skills includes all of the following components EXCEPT:
   a. Experience
   b. High salary
   c. Good judgment
   d. Confidence
10. Advanced technicians who work with quality assurance would often have which of the following included in their day-to-day responsibilities?
    a. Review of policies
    b. Collaboration with other departments
    c. Direct contact with nursing staff
    d. All of the above

CRITICAL THINKING QUESTIONS

1. You are the pharmacy technician manager for a busy pharmacy within a community setting, and your department has a job opening for an immunization technician. What would you look for in candidates for this position?
2. You have been working as a technician for over 5 years, and you want to see what type of advanced leadership roles are out there. What type of leadership skills would you want to possess to be successful in an intermediate supervisory role?

REFERENCES

Al-Sawai, A. (2013). Leadership of healthcare professionals: where do we stand? *Oman medical journal*, *28*(4), 285–287. https://doi.org/10.5001/omj.2013.79.

Corporate Finance Institute. Management Skills. Retrieved September 9. 2019 from https://corporatefinanceinstitute.com/resources/careers/soft-skills/management-skills/.

Hasan, Sarmad. Feb 2017. Top Ten Leadership Qualities That Make Good Leaders. Retrieved Sept 9, 2019 from https://blog.taskque.com/characteristics-good-leaders/.

Kohn, L. T., Corrigan, J. M., & Donaldson, M. S. (2000). *To Err is Human: Building a Safer Health System*. Washington, DC: Institute of Medicine.

Malacos, Kristy. April 17, 2016. Pharmacy Technician Leadership. Retrieved Sept 9, 2019 from https://www.pharmacytimes.com/publications/issue/2016/april2016/pharmacy-technician-leadership.

Pharmacy Technician and Education and Career Guide. Pharmacy Technician Management Roles. Retrieved September 9, 2019 from https://www.pharmacytechschools.com/pharmacy-technician-management-roles/.

Communication Within the Interdisciplinary Team

Learning Objectives

1. Define the term *interdisciplinary care team* and identify key members and their roles.
2. Discuss the necessity for interdisciplinary teamwork in today's environment.
3. Identify the benefits of a collaborate team that maintains good communication techniques.
4. Discuss strategies for advanced technicians to use to promote good communication within interdisciplinary healthcare teams.

Key Terms

Interdisciplinary care team (ICT) The team approach to treating patients physically, mentally, and spiritually through the collaborative efforts of healthcare team members and the patient.

Value-based care System where payments are based on patient outcomes; also known as *accountable care*.

Volume-based care System where incentives are based on volume and cost of care; also known as *fee-for-care service*.

INTRODUCTION

Research has shown that an **interdisciplinary care team (ICT)** approach to providing patient care allows for safer and more efficient outcomes (Fig. 4.1). The ICT is a group of healthcare professionals who work together to manage the physical, psychological, and spiritual needs of a patient. In this process, the patient is a key team member as well.

In the past, the model generally was that each healthcare professional, such as the primary care provider or physician, nurse, and pharmacist, worked independently. Each one used their expertise in the field and knowledge base to treat the patient with the aim of achieving specific outcomes. The primary care provider, such as a physician, looked at the patient with a goal of disease management and used tools related to diagnosis, surgery, or other procedures. The nurse would then follow up with management based on the primary care provider's treatment plan. This usually consisted of a rigid set of instructions, medications, or orders, and the patient was relatively uninformed of the treatment specifics. The pharmacist would provide medications prescribed by the primary care provider, and changes were made based on the instructions or orders provided. Technicians were support staff for the pharmacist and prepared medications under the pharmacist's direct supervision. For example, this individual may have been a pharmacy clerk who was trained on the job, with little input or decision-making abilities regarding the patient's care or outcomes.

NECESSITY OF INTERDISCIPLINARY TEAMWORK

Prevention and awareness are key aspects of healthcare provision today. The days of treating patients with long hospital stays and discharging them home with minimal follow-up are gone. Today, professionals use the ICT to care for the patient throughout a lifetime. This includes prevention, disease management, education, and incentives for making good lifestyle choices.

ECONOMICS

With the enactment of the Affordable Care Act, reimbursement decreases, and the increase in the cost of employers' premiums, there was a push to provide care to patients within a **value-based care** system rather than the **volume-based care** that characterized past systems. In volume-based systems, reimbursement is based on the volume of patients serviced and the number of treatments administered. For example, routine blood tests would be performed for the treatment of high blood pressure, but without the provision of patient education regarding the lifestyle changes that could help halt progression toward other, more serious conditions. There was little emphasis placed on improving overall quality of life, wellness, or disease prevention. Patients today shop for the best value for the most affordable cost, and this has created a competitive market for healthcare providers. Value-based care is a healthcare delivery system that pays based on patient health outcomes.

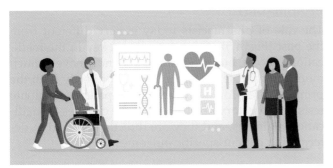

Fig. 4.1 Interdisciplinary team. (Copyright © iStock.com/elenabs.)

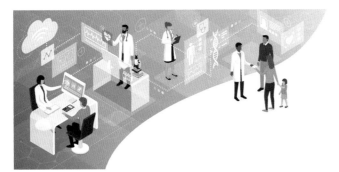

Fig. 4.2 Innovation in healthcare. (Copyright © iStock.com/elenabs.)

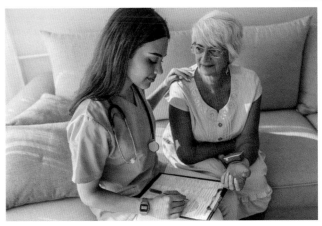

Fig. 4.3 Clinical pharmacy technician working in an advanced role taking a medication history from an elderly patient. (Copyright © iStock.com/dragana991.)

For example, many third-party insurance providers offer incentives, such as lower premiums or copays, for patient participation in exercise programs, diet control, and cessation of smoking and alcohol. These patients tend to be healthier, require less treatment, and have better management of chronic illnesses, and they are thus less costly to the company and the provider of services (Fig. 4.2).

Value-based care requires taking patients' risk factors and their engagement level in their own health into consideration. Health literacy can be described as a person's capacity or level of understanding of information in order to participate in their own health decisions. Some examples would include a patient understanding their prescription's instructions, the ability to comprehend medical education pamphlets, or negotiating a variety of physician visits. Providers are rewarded for helping patients reduce risks, improve their overall health, and live healthier lifestyles. This results in a healthier population that requires fewer tests or procedures, medications, and hospital stays. The challenge is to provide this level of care with fewer staff members and more qualified healthcare team members.

AGING POPULATION

Research shows that the average lifespan has increased. The average lifespan in North America is 81 for females and 76 for males (Statistica, 2019). This means we must care for a larger population with more illnesses and diseases and complex care requirements. It is said that the baby-boomer generation, about

70 million people, is less healthy than the previous generation (Pew Research Center, 2020). The combination of chronic conditions, such as high cholesterol, high blood pressure, diabetes, and obesity, paired with the higher life-expectancy numbers means more patients with more conditions that require treatment. Providing quality care requires an approach that includes lifestyle changes, wellness and prevention, and improved services. To meet the challenges of the healthcare needs of this huge number of patients, the interdisciplinary team approach is the best way to provide quality and efficient care (Fig. 4.3).

COMPLEXITY OF CARE REQUIREMENTS

No one healthcare team member can provide for all the complex needs of a patient. The evolution of diseases and the complexity of medications, treatments, and diagnostic testing require the healthcare professional to be more skilled and work at a higher level of knowledge. The push for continuity of care and quality improvement through organizations such as The Joint Commission requires an organization to set goals and create strategies for playing a larger role in and creating a bigger impact on every patient's health. The *2020 National Patient Safety Goals* focus on problems in healthcare safety and how to solve them. Some of the targeted areas include identification of patients, communication improvement, infection prevention, risks for patients, and surgical mistakes. See http://www.jointcommission.org/assets/1/6/2020_HAP_NPSG_goals_final.pdf for more information on these goals.

CONTINUITY OF CARE

Continuity of care is the quality of care over time. The patient, along with their healthcare team, sets a goal for high quality, cost-effective medical care. Working as a team and towards a unified goal, allows for a close relationship between patient and team and promotes better, overall health for the patient. The

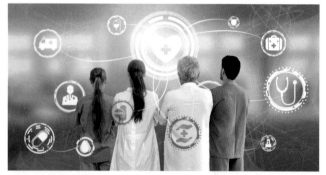

Fig. 4.4 Team members discussing a patient. (Copyright © iStock.com/NanoStockk.)

impact to the healthcare industry are significant as better quality of life means less invasive procedures, hospitalizations, or urgent care the patient needs. Ultimately the savings of these are passed to insurances and other providers of services which in turn affects every American.

This complexity of care requires either a large workforce to rally around a patient, with each one acting within that professional's scope of practice, or a team approach, with one focus and each member collaborating toward the same goal. The interdisciplinary team approach can allow for a larger impact with a smaller workforce. Many responsibilities are shared, and advanced technicians are stepping up to meet the challenges with specialty training and leadership opportunities. The once traditional roles are now blurred, and with experience and specialty training, advanced technicians can serve in many nontraditional roles (Fig. 4.4).

INTERDISCIPLINARY CARE TEAM: KEY MEMBERS AND ROLES

The ICT consists of members of each healthcare area related to the patient's needs and the patient and family members. The members function independently based on their areas of expertise, skills, and knowledge. But rather than stopping there, as in the past model, there is a continuous sharing of information among the group and collaboration toward patient-centered outcomes or goals. Each member of the ICT works together to create an effective workflow that reduces medication errors, allows for better patient satisfaction and adherence, and provides the best care delivery possible. In today's competitive healthcare environment, it is imperative for organizations to provide quality care in the most efficient way possible.

Each member of the ICT has a specific responsibility based on that individual's expertise and knowledge base. Today's patient-centered care requires all team members to perform at their highest knowledge level, and in many cases, responsibilities overlap and are shared. For example, the advanced technician can serve in a clinical role or in information technology (IT), which was traditionally a role fulfilled by a nurse or IT expert.

PHARMACIST

The role of pharmacists today is very different from the past (Fig. 4.5). Their expertise is key in the medication process, but in addition, they now have a much more clinical role. Pharmacists work directly with the primary care provider to interview patients, evaluate tests or laboratory results, and make changes to medication regimens, and they are directly involved in determining patient-specific outcomes.

ADVANCED PHARMACY TECHNICIAN

The role of the advanced technician can vary based on specialty skills or training and experience. For example, it could include a management role with a subteam of technicians who support patient goals by managing day-to-day dispensing and medication preparation, including preparing nonsterile and sterile medications (compounding). It could also be a direct clinical support member who screens test results or lab values to alert the pharmacist. Advanced technicians may also manage adverse drug reaction (ADR) programs to identify medication errors and actively work with other team members to provide solutions (Fig. 4.6).

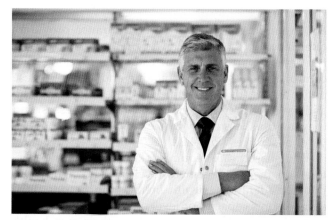

Fig. 4.5 Pharmacist in a busy hospital pharmacy. (Copyright © iStock.com/shapecharge.)

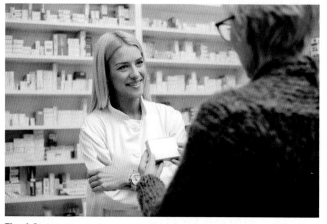

Fig. 4.6 Advanced pharmacy technician discussing an over-the-counter medication with a patient. (Copyright © iStock.com/Gligatron.)

The advanced technician team member can also be important in clinical administration roles, such as data entry of patient test results, medication changes, and reconciliation. The maintenance of accurate electronic records that are shared by the team members provides a real-time picture of the patient's current condition.

PRIMARY CARE PROVIDER

Different titles may be used for the primary care provider, such as *doctor, hospitalist,* or a specialist title related to the provider's field of expertise (e.g., *orthopedist* or *pediatrician*). The primary healthcare provider may also be another professional, this can also include other staff, such as nurse practitioners or physician's assistants. In most cases, the primary care provider leads the team in decisions for the patient based on diagnosis and a subsequent treatment plan. The team works closely to achieve the goals outlined based on the primary care provider's expertise (Fig. 4.7).

NURSE

The traditional role of the nurse as a team member consists of much more than just medication administration in today's environment. Nurses are also communicators who transfer information, through conversation and documentation, gathered from the patient directly

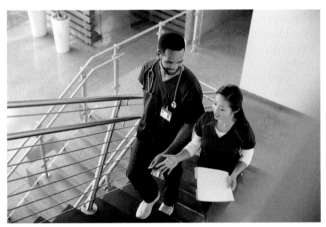

Fig. 4.7 Physician and nurse discussing the progress of a patient. (Copyright © iStock.com/monkeybusinessimages.)

to other care providers on the team. They are a direct link between the patient and other team members who are focused on the patient. Newer roles include the instructor role, which consists of teaching patients to use medical devices, such as diabetic meters or medical applications that record data. Nurses are also instrumental in medication teaching as well as monitoring of patient's clinical outcomes or functions.

PATIENT

The team includes the patient or a primary caregiver delegate for the patient. The current model for patient-centered care must include the patient in the treatment plan. The previous approach was "just do as the doctor said." In contrast, the current approach includes communication in layperson's terms about what is happening and why. For example, emoticons are used for pain-scale ratings (Fig. 4.8).

Patients are provided clear information about all tests being performed and why, medications given and what they are for, and vital sign readings.

 Tech Note

In today's typical hospital room, there is an information board, and patient care instructions are written in layperson's terms. The use of abbreviations, such as *TID, PRN, PO,* and *HS,* is avoided so that the patient can understand medication names, the last time a dose was administered, and the time when the next dose is due.

Patients are encouraged to participate in their own care and in the decision-making process through education and instruction. This goes far beyond just the care provided during an event or for the immediate condition being treated. For example, in chronic illnesses such as diabetes, chronic obstructive pulmonary disease (COPD), and heart disease, education regarding diet, lifestyle choices, and prevention is key to keeping the patient well and providing the best quality of life. The care doesn't just stop with the patient's discharge. This also allows for better adherence

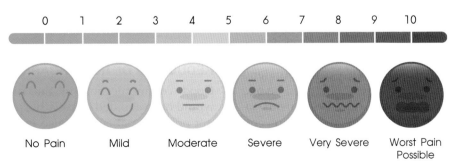

Fig. 4.8 Pain scale. (Copyright © iStock.com/anuwat-meereewee.)

to medication regimens, less repeat hospitalizations, and fewer repeat visits for physicians.

SUPPORT PERSONNEL

The additional key members of the interdisciplinary team can vary depending on disease states and various practice settings, such as home care, long-term care facilities, hospice, assisted living, clinics, physician offices, and community pharmacies. Common support personnel include medical assistants (MAs), laboratory and radiology technicians (RTs), certified nurse technicians (CNAs), dietary personnel, and clerical and administrative staff.

There are also coordinating efforts through other departments, which might involve case managers, social workers, and transfer facility representatives for those requiring long-term care. These support team members serve to work toward continuous care and can also include advanced technicians in roles involving discharge planning and medication adherence programs.

BENEFITS OF GOOD COMMUNICATION FOR THE INTERDISCIPLINARY TEAM

To maintain a strong team, each member must be aligned with the patient goals, which are established through a collaborative process. This process must include clear communication among all members. Goals must be established that ensure every action works in conjunction with another and that duplication of services is reduced as much as possible. There are several benefits of good communication among the members of the ICT that relate to the providers and the patients.

BENEFITS FOR SOCIETY

Good communication within an interdisciplinary team allows for better overall health for the patient, which creates a healthier population in general. This reduces healthcare costs and lost work time, thus benefiting the overall economy. Treating a patient through awareness, incentives for healthier lifestyle choices, and affordable premiums for both employers and employees supports a strong economic base for society.

IMPROVED PATIENT SATISFACTION

Patient satisfaction can make a huge difference. Good communication among the ICT demonstrates a collaborative and quality approach in treating the patient. Patients view duplication of services or repetition of basic questions as disorganized and poor service provision. The challenge to include patients in their own care can be hindered greatly if they are not confident in the team's approach to their care and well-being. A lack of confidence in the ICT can lead patients to avoid participation in wellness and disease prevention activities and cause excessive emergency visits or additional costly tests or procedures, which affect the patient's health negatively and should be avoided.

Patient satisfaction can be improved with simple acts, such as making a call to a pharmacy with special instructions, providing additional notes or documentation, or working with a designated patient's family member.

Case Study

A 76-year-old patient is admitted with a diabetic episode. The patient was recently diagnosed with diabetes and placed on insulin by his physician. He was instructed by the physician's nurse to pick up a meter at the pharmacy and check his glucose levels daily.

During the patient admission interview and medication history, the advanced technician asks, "How often do you check your blood sugar, Mr. Davis?" He replies, "I got a meter but never really was told how to use it, so my granddaughter has been coming once a week and checking it for me." The technician checks the notes in the record and sees an entry from the nurse at the doctor's office. It states, "Patient to pick up a blood glucose meter at the pharmacy, and patient was told he would get instructions there." She pulls the original prescription to see if it has instructions or a notation regarding the pharmacy teaching requirement. It doesn't note anything other than the prescription for the meter, strips, and lancets.

Could this hospital visit have been avoided? Would better communication have made a difference?

The nurse assumed that the patient clearly understood her instructions. The pharmacy also neglected to teach the patient how to use the meter. The pharmacy assumed the physician's office had provided instructions because the patient didn't ask for any.

Good communication within the ICT could have avoided this visit. For example, the prescription could have included wording regarding "patient instructions required" to alert the pharmacy of the need to provide patient education. Both the pharmacy and nurse assumed the other would teach the patient. The consequences of poor communication in this case are that the patient will experience a setback in health, several providers will have to pay for the care, and the patient's confidence level in his treatment will be decreased. All of this could have been avoided with some simple good communication.

 Tech Note

Generally, with higher levels of collaboration and better communication techniques, the risk of negative patient outcomes is reduced.

REDUCTION OF HEALTHCARE COSTS

Good communication in the previous case study would have avoided a costly hospital stay. This affects not only the patient but also every person receiving healthcare benefits. Effective communication can reduce duplication of services, length of stay in facilities, and additional episodes in the future. Wasted nurse and physician time is extremely costly, and these costs affect the whole healthcare and provider payment system. The use of good communication among an ICT creates an efficient and quality-based approach to care for the patient. The constant flow of information between the providers and team members allows real-time data for every caregiver involved with the patient.

STRATEGIES FOR PROMOTING GOOD ICT COMMUNICATION

Advanced technicians with experience and specialty training can be a significant part of the team. An ICT can be dedicated to a particular type of care or managed in a separate area and often includes technicians who serve in clinical or operational roles along- other team members. This increases efficiency and the level of care that can be offered.

USE OF DECENTRALIZED PHARMACIES (SATELLITES)

About 80% of today's hospitals use satellite pharmacies, or pharmacies outside the main pharmacy. These are usually staffed with a pharmacist and advanced technicians who have additional experience or training in the particular area. For example, some hospitals have chemotherapy units where certified compounded sterile preparation technicians (CSPTs) or advanced trained technicians prepare all cancer medications in a separate US Pharmacopeia (USP) "800" facility. This allows a direct communication channel between the nurses who are administering medications, the patient receiving the medications, the physician, and the pharmacist. This also reduces delay times in administration because the decentralized pharmacy is on the floor alongside the patient rooms and nurse's unit.

USE OF TECHNOLOGY

Communication with team members through discussions, documentation, and electronic records is an important element of the care process. Advanced technicians who have strong skills in data entry, data analysis, and clerical or administrative work are key members of ICTs. Sharing data and recording results in anticipation of treatment reviews or possible changes can increase delivery time and reduce errors (Fig. 4.9).

COLLABORATION EFFORTS AND COMMUNICATION

Collaboration involves taking the time to meet regularly and working with other committees or stakeholders that affect system or organizational goals to promote quality care and employee satisfaction. Encouraging open discussion to brainstorm ideas allows the team to work through problems and find solutions. Asking questions and challenging oneself

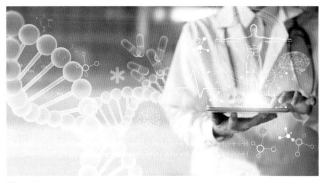

Fig. 4.9 Today's healthcare environment includes many forms of technology. (Copyright © iStock.com/ipopba.)

to work through situations by communicating with others make the team stronger. Advanced technicians often act as liasons between other departments by serving on committees or participating in quality improvement programs. The advanced technician's use of experience and advanced training or specialty certifications brings a different perspective to the group and improves the services the facility is able to offer.

Advanced technicians are serving in clinical, administrative, quality control, medication safety, and specialty roles as part of today's ICT. A successful team requires all members to work toward their highest level of expertise in skills, knowledge, and communication. The overall goals are patient centered in a value-based system, which is today's healthcare model. Good communication and efficiency are key for patient satisfaction, positive treatment outcomes, and the ability to be competitive in today's healthcare environment. As more specialty technician certifications are established and organizations seek advanced technicians who have leadership and management skills, patient care will continue to benefit, which will result in better health for a higher proportion of the population.

REVIEW QUESTIONS

1. Which of the following best describes value-based care?
   a. Providers pay based on accountable milestones.
   b. Providers pay a fee for each service.
   c. Providers pay based on current healthcare costs.
   d. Providers pay based on disease states.
2. Which of the following best describes volume-based care?
   a. Providers pay based on accountable milestones.
   b. Providers pay a fee for each service.
   c. Providers pay based on current healthcare costs.
   d. Providers pay based on disease states.
3. Which aspects of patient care are involved when applying an ICT approach?
   a. Mental
   b. Physical
   c. Spiritual
   d. All of the above

4. Before the ICT approach, which health care professional used diagnostic testing, surgeries, or other procedures to provide the nurses with the next step in the patient's care?
   a. Physician
   b. Nurse
   c. Pharmacist
   d. Pharmacy technician

5. According to Statistica, what is the average lifespan for women in North America?
   a. 81 years
   b. 76 years
   c. 65 years
   d. 75 years

6. According to Statistica, what is the average lifespan for men in North America?
   a. 76 years
   b. 81 years
   c. 65 years
   d. 79 years

7. What percentage of pharmacies use satellites or decentralized pharmacies today?
   a. 80%
   b. 75%
   c. 50%
   d. 25%

8. In which areas do advanced pharmacy technicians currently have roles?
   a. Clinical administration
   b. Medication safety

   c. Information technology
   d. All of the above

9. All of the following are considered chronic illnesses EXCEPT:
   a. Cancer
   b. Diabetes
   c. COPD
   d. High cholesterol

10. Which of the following can be used in the patient-centered care model to maintain the best quality of life for a patient?
    a. Diet education
    b. Change in lifestyle choices
    c. Immunizations
    d. All of the above

CRITICAL THINKING QUESTIONS

1. A patient presents to the pharmacy with a new prescription for a cholesterol-lowering medication. He is obese and smokes a pack of cigarettes a day. Along with the filling of the mediation and provision of instructions, what other steps would be appropriate for the patient to manage this condition?

2. You want to apply for a new position as a clinical technician at a large hospital. This position involves reviewing patient laboratory results for blood-clotting times each morning. What type of communication skills would be necessary for this job?

REFERENCES

Chen, A. M., Kiersma, M. E., Keib, C. N., & Cailor, S. (2015). *Fostering Interdisciplinary Communication between Pharmacy and Nursing Students. American journal of pharmaceutical education*, 79(6), 83. https://doi.org/10.5688/ajpe79683.

CRXADMIN. *Collaboration and communication: The role pharmacists play in nurse satisfaction.* Retrieved September 26, 2019 from https://www.completerx.com/collaboration-and-communication-the-role-pharmacists-play-in-nurse-satisfaction/.

Nancarrow, S. A., Booth, A., Ariss, S., Smith, T., Enderby, P., & Roots, A. (2013). *Ten principles of good interdisciplinary teamwork. Human resources for health*, 11. https://doi.org/10.1186/1478-4491-11-19.

Pew Research Center, *Millennials Overtake Baby Boomers as America's Largest Generation*, April 2020. Retrieved July 21, 2020 from https://www.pewresearch.org/fact-tank/2020/04/28/millennials-overtake-baby-boomers-as-americas-largest-generation/.

Statistica. *Average Life Expectancy in North America for those Born in 2019, by gender and Region.* Retrieved September 25, 2019 from https://www.statista.com/statistics/274513/life-expectancy-in-north-america/.

Operational Functions

5

Learning Objectives

1. Discuss the use of advanced technicians in pharmacy workflow processes and the daily operations of a pharmacy.
2. Discuss how the use of advanced technicians in operational roles benefits the patient-centered model and organizations.

3. List some operational functions for advanced technicians in today's pharmacy.

Key Terms

Analytics The discovery, interpretation, and communication of meaningful patterns in data.
Comorbid The presence of two chronic diseases or conditions at the same time.
Patient adherence program Method used for patients to follow medication, treatments, lifestyle, or self-directed regimens in order to stay healthy.

Patient-centered model A team approach in providing care for patients that includes all parties sharing information and assisting the patient in prevention and ongoing care.
Value-based care System based on accountability, in which payments for services are based on outcomes rather than volume.

INTRODUCTION

With the complexity of healthcare and declining reimbursements, pharmacies must operate as efficiently as possible to stay competitive while providing the highest quality of care. This includes the use of advanced technicians in many operational roles to support the organization's mission. Traditionally, technicians served in dispensing or customer service roles, such as clerks or cashiers. Today's pharmacy has evolved to be a more **patient-centered model** and must serve patients using the **value-based care** model (Fig. 5.1). The focus is providing patients with the best and safest care while setting goals that include accountable outcomes for their own health. This requires every pharmacy team member to work cohesively and integrate services with other healthcare providers, and the model includes wellness and disease management along with medications.

BENEFITS OF USING ADVANCED TECHNICIANS IN PHARMACY OPERATIONS

The American Society of Health-System Pharmacists (ASHP) Practice Advancement Initiative (PAI) discusses optimizing the role of pharmacy technicians to achieve patient goals and advance their health needs. As part of the initiative, the following challenges are included

concerning the use of advanced technicians in patient care (ASHP, 2015):

- Encourage technicians to actively perform all traditional preparation and distribution activities.
- Encourage technicians to handle nontraditional and advanced responsibilities to allow more time for pharmacists to participate in direct patient care.
- Promote standardized training and certification requirements for advanced technician roles.

The PAI supports using the advanced technician in operational functions such as dispensing, preparation, and other day-to-day operations to allow the pharmacist to be as involved as possible in every aspect of the patient's treatment. Disease prevention and awareness are key areas for all healthcare providers today, and the pharmacy plays a vital role in efforts in these areas. The operational benefits and cost reductions can be seen in simple workflow processes, such as movement or steps required, optimal scheduling, assignment of tasks to key personnel, and the use of technology and informatics tools.

 Tech Note

Six Sigma is a common industry standard used to increase the efficiency of organizations by identifying processes that can improve workflow (Fig. 5.2).

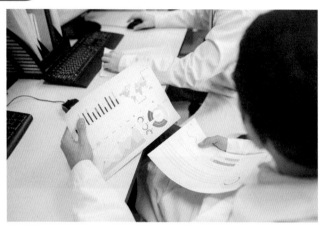

Fig. 5.1 Technician analyzing operational data. (Copyright © iStock.com/SeventyFour.)

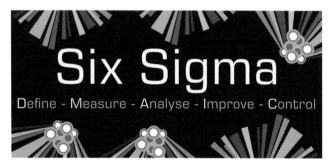

Fig. 5.2 Six Sigma. (Copyright © iStock.com/ileezhun.)

PROCESS IMPROVEMENT

Six Sigma is a process that incorporates six steps to determine efficiency and help improve methods once data have been collected. Many organizations use this method to increase efficiency, make improvements, and evaluate continuously to improve quality. The Six Sigma process includes defining the goal, measuring the processes used, analyzing the data, designing changes to meet the goal, and verifying that the plan will meet the defined needs.

One of the most important Six Sigma processes is to evaluate workspace and the number of steps or amount of motion a task requires. Technicians in advanced roles can be instrumental in evaluating current processes and making suggestions for improvements in the areas they oversee. For example, if a task is to reach into a bin and remove a medication to be placed in another container, the distance between the two containers must be traveled. If this space is too large, the task involves excessive movement, which takes up time and energy. The placement of items, furniture, and shelving should be considered when thinking through each task. Improving productivity increases the amount of work that can be done efficiently. The goal is to reduce motion and travel time. Another consideration is the movement of medications from one area to another (Fig. 5.3).

MOVEMENT (WORKFLOW PROCESSES)

Workflow is very important is completing tasks efficiently and quickly. In a community pharmacy, this

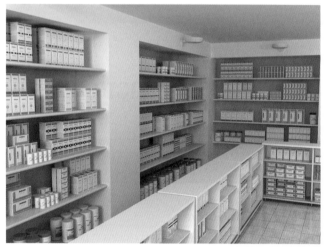

Fig. 5.3 Pharmacy layout. Stocked shelves with work counter close by. (Copyright © iStock.com/cosinart.)

includes the placement of different work areas such as drive thru window, front counter, dispensing areas, compounding areas, and spaces for confidential communications such as patient or physician calls.

Proper workflow and use of space will benefit workers because they can complete tasks easier and spend their time on other tasks rather than movement inside large spaces. Workflow and space improvements benefit patients because services can be rendered faster and more efficiently in a system where tasks can be completed easily and quickly. Another benefit is that space is used more efficiently, so less space is needed overall, which is an economic benefit. In addition, using advanced technicians in these areas helps to manage workflow and make use of their expertise. A lead technician dedicated to an area or specialty in the department sees the day-to-day activities and can arrange space and tasks and collaborate with others to allow for a seamless transition or movement of medications and supplies between areas (Fig. 5.4).

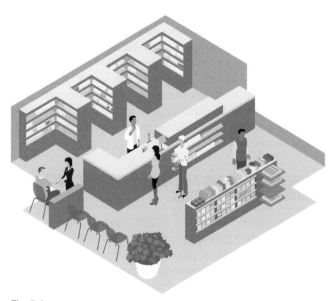

Fig. 5.4 Community pharmacy layout. (Copyright © iStock.com/mathisworks.)

Case Study

As the lead in the hospital pharmacy area that is responsible for unit-dose (UD) stock medications that are dispensed through an automated dispensing cabinet (ADC), how would you arrange the following items and areas?

Area 1: Repackaging Area

    Bulk stock

    Supplies for repackaging (blisters, gloves, labeling stock)

    Area used for repackaging (printer, counter, etc.)

Area 2: ADC delivery/check area

    Bins for UD medication supply

    Bags for packaging

The repackaging area or preparation area should be small, and each supply should be located adjacent to the next one in the process. Move the work closer to the worker in general. Place the stock bottle shelving close to the working space and supplies that are needed to prepare the UD medications. The final product should be placed close to the next section or area so that the flow moves easily and quickly to the final destination, which in this case is the area where the prepared UD medications are kept.

For the ADC delivery/check area, the person responsible for maintaining the UD stock area should be able to maintain stocked bins and pull these medications easily for delivery to the ADCs. The bins should be alphabetically arranged and close to the packaging (bags) supplies and delivery cart(s). An area designated for verification by the pharmacist should be located close to the delivery carts.

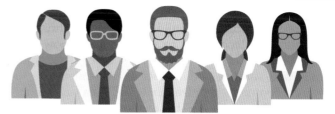

Fig. 5.5 Pharmacy staff. (Copyright © iStock.com/aelitta.)

month and the following week? Or consider the time of year for a busy pharmacy with a wellness clinic staffed by an advanced technician and a pharmacist. Wouldn't it be appropriate to have extra staffing during the flu season to accommodate immunizations?

Each state has its own regulations regarding ratios of pharmacists to technicians. When hiring or staffing a department, this ratio must be considered. As an advanced technician serving in a leadership role, you may be tasked with serving on a hiring committee or reassigning personnel to meet this ratio. In a large healthcare system such as a hospital, there may be satellites or outlying clinics that are staffed independently from one another (Fig. 5.5).

 Tech Note

Most pharmacies have a "fast movers" section that holds the medications or products that are dispensed most often. This allows staff the quickest access to these items, which saves time because they are used so often.

ADVANCED TECHNICIAN ROLE IN SCHEDULING AND ASSIGNMENT OF TASKS

In today's healthcare environment, achieving cost reduction while providing the highest-quality patient care is a struggle. Determining technicians' strengths and ensuring they are able to use their advanced knowledge base and training promotes a maximum level of efficiency. As pharmacies continue to change and advanced technicians take on more responsibilities, there are more opportunities for management or lead positions as schedulers. Understanding the correlation between the volume of work and certain days, months, and seasons, for example, is key to maintaining efficiency in every circumstance. A lead who works directly in dispensing areas, for example, is well positioned to provide guidance on which days to have extra staffing. For example, the busiest time for a community pharmacy is usually the first of each month. Would it make sense to be short staffed on the 31st and the week thereafter and overstaffed on the 22nd of the

Case Study

The cancer center of a big hospital system has its own technicians and pharmacist who regularly work there. One of the technicians is going on maternity leave in about 3 months, and as the scheduler, you have to assign someone to cover the time she is out. During her time off, not only should the pharmacy match the state ratio of 3 technicians to 1 pharmacist, with at least two of them being certified pharmacy technicians (CPhTs), but the fill-in employee must be trained in sterile hazardous preparation.

You have two choices, as follows:

- One CPhT works in the intravenous (IV) room and has specialty training in hazardous preparation as well. She is your best advanced technician for IV lines, and the area is really busy.
- Another CPhT has worked in the IV room recently but needs a little refresher course on hazardous preparation. She is currently rotating between the UD area and the IV room as needed.

The CPhT who just needs a refresher would be the most appropriate choice. This CPhT could be trained internally by the current technician, attend an outside specialty course, or become a certified compounded sterile preparation technician (CSPT). This would give the CPhT an opportunity to advance her skills, and the pharmacy would have another advanced technician with specialty training in hazardous preparation as backup. If the more experienced CPhT were pulled from the busy IV room to fill in, that area would not be as efficient, thus slowing down productivity for the whole department. This is turn would affect other departments and, ultimately, the patient.

As discussed in Chapter 3, being a good leader includes supporting and building up other technicians. Encouraging technicians to advance their knowledge and skills provides a better pool of staff to fill necessary roles and support one another as team members toward a common organizational goal. As a lead technician scheduler, rotating staff to allow for cross-training helps to maintain the workflow with minimal disruption. Disruptions can occur just from certain people going to lunch at the worst time! In the scenario in the previous case study, for example, letting the main IV technician go to lunch without a qualified technician to cover the time could cause an avalanche of backorders that snowballs for the rest of the day.

ADVANCED TECHNICIANS AND THE USE OF TECHNOLOGY AND INFORMATICS IN OPERATIONS

The daily operational functions of today's pharmacy must include automation and the use of informatics (Fig. 5.6). Sharing patient information across healthcare team members is necessary for the patient-centered model. The patient's electronic health record (EHR) is part of every aspect of patient treatment today, from the primary care provider's process of check-in to ongoing medication reconciliation and adherence programs. Clinical skills are needed to use such systems, as discussed later, but the operational functions require an advanced understanding of technology to store and maintain this flow of information. Advanced technicians serving in an informatics role will be challenged in the workflow or communication stream as it moves through the department and outside to other areas. Much like the Six Sigma process for "movement" discussed earlier, the flow of information must travel the shortest distance and to the correct staff in the most appropriate order. This is a challenge in every organization, and the bigger the organization, the greater the challenge. Ramifications for patients and their safety must also be considered. Making a mistake on a memo regarding someone's contact information will not have the same ramifications as making a mistake in the name or amount of a medication.

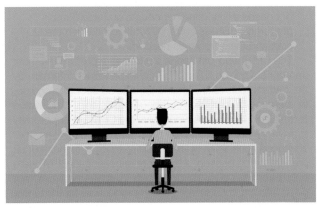

Fig. 5.6 Business analysis. (Copyright © iStock.com/TCmake_photo.)

Operational functions must include safeguards and checks to establish that information is being disseminated correctly and to only those allowed to view it, as mandated by the Health Insurance Portability and Accountability Act (HIPAA). An advanced technician who has a good understanding of how information is exchanged within the department and with others who provide patient services is positioned to deliver the highest quality of care provided in the most efficient manner.

There are many automated dispensing systems in use today. This has created a much higher level of efficiency than could have been achieved in the past. Such systems give the pharmacist more time to participate in patient counseling and adherence programs. Advanced technicians often manage automated dispensing areas, and in some states, they perform "tech check tech" (TCT) procedures. TCT is the process of an advanced technician checking the work of another technician in the preparation of UD medications or the filling of ADC in institutional or hospital settings. Each state board regulates TCT, and in some states, there are added responsibilities. Distributing the workload to include checks at the advanced technician level has been shown to decrease medication errors. For example, the University of Wisconsin Hospital and Clinics implemented a TCT program and recorded an accuracy rate of greater than 99.8% for technicians filling UD medication cassettes (Reed et al., 2011). This level of accuracy and responsibility through the use of technology increases the amount of services the organization can provide. It is also a benefit for the organization because more work can be done with less staffing, which directly affects budgets.

 Tech Note

There are 17 states (California, Colorado, Idaho, Iowa, Kansas, Kentucky, Illinois, Michigan, Minnesota, Montana, North Dakota, North Carolina, Maryland, South Carolina, Ohio, Oregon, and Washington) that allow pharmacy technicians to check the work of other technicians in hospital and institutional or community settings (National Association of Boards of Pharmacy [NABP], 2009) (Fig. 5.7).

ADVANCED TECHNICIANS IN BUSINESS SYSTEM ANALYTICS AND DATA ANALYSIS

Operational functions depend on a continuous process of data analysis and process improvements. Advanced technicians often serve in lead roles in collecting operational, safety, and clinical information. **Analytics** is the process of finding data or information and evaluating it for patterns. Once the data or information has been evaluated, it can then be used to create process improvement plans and shared with the team. Having critical thinking skills and being able to filter what is needed

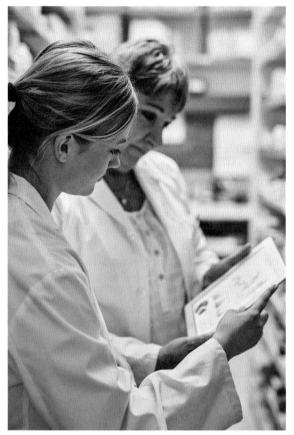

Fig. 5.7 Advanced pharmacy technician verifying the technician's work. (Copyright © iStock.com/PeopleImages.)

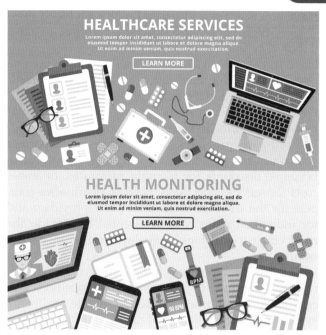

Fig. 5.8 Healthcare services and monitoring. (Copyright © iStock.com/Jane_Kelly.)

from what is available are valuable skills for advanced technicians who wish to fulfill this role. They also may streamline information flows, develop reports to share within the organization, create processes for implementation in an area that is inefficient, or implement a cost-saving measure. Often, they are asked to collaborate with committees, such as the Pharmacy and Therapeutics (P&T) Committee and committees for medication safety, infusion services, or purchasing. Sharing the information and discussing the potential pitfalls can lead to gathering data to create optimal practices.

Business analytics can also include working with third-party providers and streamlining payment of services from third parties or other payer sources. This effort involves ongoing observation and gathering of results or data to use for improvements in the practices of an organization, as discussed in Chapter 9.

BENEFITS OF USING ADVANCED TECHNICIANS IN THE PATIENT-CENTERED MODEL

The patient-centered model is based on the value-based system, which centers around patient outcomes and adherence to programs, testing, and medication regimens (Fig. 5.8). Patients are encouraged to maintain healthy lifestyles through education, awareness, and everyday activities as part of

a **patient adherence program**. Self-monitoring of activities such as smoking and alcohol consumption is encouraged and reported through self-surveys on a yearly basis. Patient adherence is the degree to which a patient follows guidelines for medication, therapy, lifestyle, or self-directed programs, such as exercise or lifestyle regimens. Employers support the patient adherence model by enacting the self-surveys for employees and offering training or classes on healthy choices.

Some common questions found on an employee survey can include the following:
What is your height, weight, waist size, and body mass index (BMI)?
How many servings of **trans fat** do you have per week?
How many servings of whole grains do you have per week?
How many servings of refined grains do you have per week?
How many alcoholic drinks do you have per week?
How many servings of red meat do you have per week?
How many servings of fish do you have per week?
How many servings of dairy do you have per week?
Do you use tobacco products?
Do you have at least $1000 in a savings account?
Do you take time for yourself?
Do you have someone to discuss problems with?
How many sugar-sweetened soft drinks do you drink per week?
Do you look forward to coming to work?
How many hours do you sleep at night?
Do you get out of breath from walking two blocks?
Do you have pain in your knees after walking two blocks or climbing stairs?

Have you ever been diagnosed with high blood pressure, high cholesterol, diabetes, arthritis, irritable bowel syndrome, or Crohn's disease?

Have you ever been prescribed medications or are you currently taking medication for any of the chronic diseases listed in the previous question?

Do you ride a bicycle or motorcycle?

How many hours do you spend outdoors each week?

Third-party providers offer incentives to the partner companies and patients, such as less costly gym memberships, discounts for monthly premiums, or lower costs for services and plans. Because pharmacies compete for the contracts from third-party providers and for individual patients, it is essential to provide the most efficient and highest-quality services to remain competitive.

The use of advanced technicians in operational roles will continue to grow as specialty positions and certifications continue to be added. As the healthcare system faces the challenges of caring for older patients with **comorbid** diseases, the number of patients using counseling, medication regimens, and treatments will increase. Ventures by Amazon and other companies that are traditionally not associated with healthcare (Fig. 5.9) into wellness and pharmacy, combining with newer value-based reimbursement models, are providing even more opportunities for highly trained professionals such as advanced technicians. In addition, for providers to be able to offer employer and employee discounts and supportive incentives, pharmacies must operate with cost-effective measures while continuing to provide care of the highest quality. This includes proper staffing, proper assignment of roles, and the use of advanced technicians in operational functions such as data analysis and staffing, which allow an organization to stay competitive and offer better choices.

> ### 💬 Tech Note
>
> It is better to work smart than to work hard. The use of advanced technicians with knowledge and experience is one of the best ways to work smart.

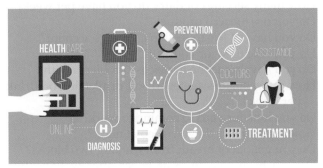

Fig. 5.9 Medicine and technology. (Copyright © iStock.com/elenabs.)

REVIEW QUESTIONS

1. Which of the following is NOT a type of incentive offered in a value-based care system?
   a. Discounted employee premiums
   b. Discounted prescription plans
   c. Gym membership coupons
   d. Discount for seeing primary care provider monthly

2. Which method is used to increase the efficiency of organizations by identifying processes that can improve workflow?
   a. API
   b. Six Sigma
   c. Value-based care
   d. Volume-based care

3. Which of the following is an advantage of proper staffing that uses advanced technicians?
   a. Fewer errors
   b. Higher quality of services
   c. Cost-effectiveness
   d. All of the above

4. The University of Wisconsin Hospital and Clinics implemented a TCT program and recorded which accuracy rate for technicians filling UD medication cassettes?
   a. >99.8%
   b. >75%
   c. <99.8%
   d. <75%

5. Which number of technicians, out of 10 currently available, would be most appropriate for staffing on the second day of the month in a community setting?
   a. 10
   b. 5
   c. 3
   d. 7

6. How many states, as of 2009, allow TCT?
   a. 17
   b. 12
   c. 22
   d. 9

7. All of the following states allow TCT EXCEPT:
   a. South Carolina
   b. North Carolina
   c. Indiana
   d. Maryland

8. Which committee might an advanced technician with expanded roles serve on?
   a. P&T
   b. Infusion services committee
   c. Medication safety committee
   d. All of the above

9. What type of information might be gathered during the self-evaluation for third-party providers?
   a. Current medications
   b. Eating habits

c. Amount of regular exercise

d. All of the above

10. What type of disease or condition could be indicated by a patient who notes the issue of "excessive urination" on a self-evaluation?

a. Prostate problems

b. Diabetes

c. COPD

d. Both a and b

11. What type of diseases or conditions could be indicated by a patient who notes, "I spend less than 1 hour a day in direct sunlight" on a self-evaluation?

a. Depression

b. Vitamin D deficiency

c. Anemia

d. Both a and b

CRITICAL THINKING QUESTIONS

1. As a lead technician in a busy hospital, you are tasked with creating a process-improvement plan for your area. Identify at least three of the Six Sigma steps you should incorporate into the plan.

2. Name at least two ways you could improve the following situation using the knowledge you have gained regarding movement and workflow: The space used for overstock for the IV room is located in the back of the pharmacy, and items are just dropped off at the back door and not organized very well on the available shelving. To gather stock, you must walk through the entire area to find what you need. The area where pickup/deliveries are kept is on the opposite side of the room from both the IV room and the overstock area.

REFERENCES

American Society of Health-System Pharmacists (ASHP). (2015). *Practice Advancement Initiative*. Retrieved October 24, 2019 from https://www.ashp.org/-/media/assets/pharmacy.

American Society of Health-System Pharmacists (ASHP). Retrieved October 23, 2019 from https://www. ashp.org/Pharmacy-Technician/About-Pharmacy-Technicians/Advanced-Pharmacy-Technician-Roles/Business-Systems-Analyst.

Reed, M., Thomley, S., Ludwig, B., & Rough, S. (2011). Experience with a "tech-check-tech" program in an academic medical center. *American Journal of Health-System Pharmacy, 68*(19), 1820–1823.

6 Technology and Dispensing Systems

Learning Objectives

1. Discuss how the five rights of medication administration safety are achieved using automated dispensing technology.
2. Discuss how the use of automated dispensing systems and advanced technology can benefit today's pharmacy.
3. Discuss remote pharmacy and the use of advanced technicians as support.
4. List ways advanced technicians can be used as support in the use of technology and automated dispensing systems.

Key Terms

Automated dispensing cabinet (ADC) Electronic cabinet used to dispense supplies or medications.

Automated dispensing devices (ADDs) Electronic devices used to dispense items such as medications or supplies.

Barcode medication administration (BCMA) Tracking and dispensing system that uses the barcodes found on products.

Computerized physician order entry (CPOE) Process of electronic entry of physician orders.

Electronic health record (EHR) A patient's complete medical record, including medications and treatment plan.

Electronic medication administration record (eMAR) A patient's medication record that is kept electronically.

Periodic automatic replenishment (PAR) level Expected number of items kept on hand at a given time.

Radiofrequency identification (RFID) tags Tags used on medications or supplies to transmit data about an item through radio waves to the antenna/reader combination.

INTRODUCTION

Today's pharmacy must embrace technology to increase efficiency as the use of clinical pharmacy services increases (Fig. 6.1). With advances in medical technology comes a longer life expectancy, but this longer lifespan often includes many complicated medical conditions. Automated dispensing systems, virtual dispensing, and remote pharmacy are just some of the common practices in which trained technicians can be used in advanced leadership roles. A medication error can lead to extended stays in institutional facilities, which is costly to providers and patients. Automated systems include safeguards for managing medications and preventing errors or drug mishaps.

PATIENT SAFETY CONSIDERATIONS ENHANCED THROUGH THE USE OF AUTOMATED DISPENSING SYSTEMS

Medication management strategies such as automated dispensing and reconciliation are commonly used in today's pharmacy practice. The advanced technician serves in a support role in the use of these strategies. The overall goal is to provide the safest and most efficient care delivered by the most qualified staff. The five rights of medication administration have been applied for years, but with advances in technology, these have been enhanced.

 Tech Note

Pharmacies must deliver the highest levels of patient safety at the lowest possible cost (Fig. 6.2).

THE FIVE RIGHTS OF MEDICATION ADMINISTRATION

The manual ways of determining the five rights of medication administration—right patient, right medication, right time, right route, and right dose—involve some simple practices, such as the use of open-ended questions to ensure the right patient. In this approach, verification of a patient includes questions that force the recipient to answer with something other than *yes* or *no*—for example, "What is your name or address?" rather than "Is your address 123 Brown Street" or "Is your name Ms. Davis?"

However, patients are often distracted and do not really hear the questions asked. This could be because of pain or trauma for a hospital patient; a previous situation, such as the information learned in a doctor's office visit; or the presence of children or other family members. Distracted patients may acknowledge parts of a conversation that they really didn't hear or assume things that weren't discussed. Thus, for right route and time, visual inspection by the preparer or technician and then verification by the pharmacist are commonly used in manual verification systems.

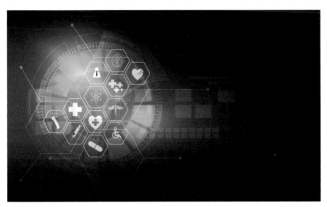

Fig. 6.1 Medicine technology (Copyright © iStock.com/ Panuwat-Sikham.)

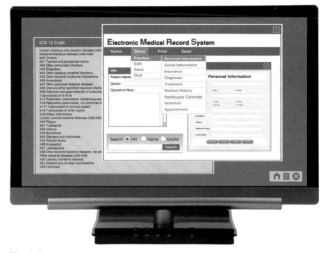

Fig. 6.3 Sample electronic health record. (Copyright © iStock.com/ pandpstock001.)

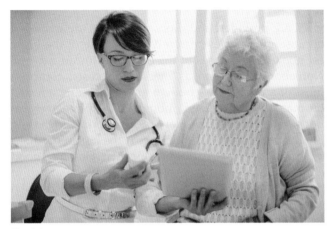

Fig. 6.2 Pharmacy technician consulting with a patient. (Copyright © iStock.com/Eva-Katalin.)

There is an additional layer of verification offered by the use of automated dispensing technology in the inpatient setting, in which a patient is verified by the use of a three-way check system. The nurse scans his or her badge to identify the administration staff. Next, the patient's armband with a barcode specific to the patient is scanned. This verifies electronically that the person administering the medication is documented, as is the patient receiving the medication. The system stores this medication information and records it in the patient's **electronic medication administration record (eMAR)** in real time; the eMAR can then be reviewed by other supporting staff participating in the patient's care. The **electronic health record (EHR)** incorporates the eMAR information and is the electronic version of the patient's chart. The EHR contains information regarding conditions and a history of medications, tests, and other measures used to treat the patient (Fig. 6.3). Both the eMAR and the EHR will be used by the advanced technician and pharmacist to maintain a complete and current record of the patient's health and medication history.

USING ADVANCED TECHNOLOGY TO IDENTIFY RIGHT MEDICATION

For verification of the right drug and dose, it was common to review the printed prescription label against the stock bottle through a visual inspection. The technology available today still involves a visual inspection but adds the use of barcodes, **radiofrequency identification (RFID) tags,** or the medication's National Drug Code (NDC) numbers.

The NDC number is a series of 10 digits used to identify a medication. It contains three parts: labeler, product, and package (Fig. 6.4).

RFID numbers were traditionally used in warehouses to identify products, and the US Food and Drug Administration (FDA) now supports the use of RFID tags as a method of tracking products in the healthcare environment. A unique number is assigned by the manufacturer, and any future transactions or movements of that product can be traced. This is especially useful in the tracking of controlled substances in the ongoing effort to thwart abuse.

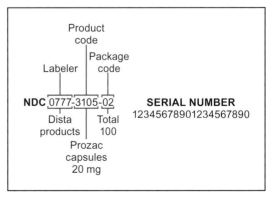

Fig. 6.4 Example of a National Drug Code (NDC) number broken down by section. (From Davis, K., & Guerra, A. [2019]. *Mosby's pharmacy technician* [5th ed.]. St. Louis, MO: Elsevier.)

Fig. 6.5 Example barcode label. (Copyright © iStock.com/LordRuner.)

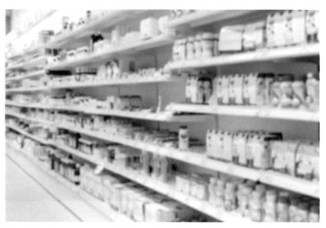

Fig. 6.7 Pharmacy stock. (Copyright © iStock.com/kjekol.)

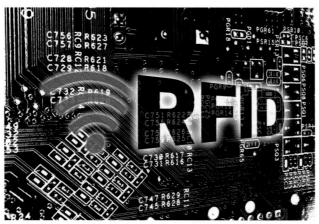

Fig. 6.6 Example of radiofrequency identification (RFID). (Copyright © iStock.com/8vFanl.)

 Tech Note

Large companies are participating in the FDA's efforts to use RFID codes, including Abbott Laboratories, Barr Pharmaceuticals, Cardinal Health, CVS, Johnson & Johnson, McKesson, Pfizer, Procter & Gamble, and Walmart (Brewin, 2004). Others include Amerisource-Bergan and Walgreens.

In addition to the tracking benefit, RFID allows for real-time information that is available to all healthcare providers or related agencies. Barcodes use readers to process a single piece of information (Fig. 6.5). RFID technology sends large amounts of information through radio waves, which can be acquired and shared automatically (Fig. 6.6).

BENEFITS OF AUTOMATED DISPENSING SYSTEMS AND TECHNOLOGY FOR TODAY'S PHARMACY

With the use of automated dispensing systems comes added benefits for the pharmacy and today's healthcare industry. There must be an improvement in the way services are provided and daily operations are managed because pharmacies currently have some of the highest nonlabor expenses in the entire healthcare system. Nonlabor costs, such as medication costs, comprise most of a pharmacy's budget and are greatly affected by managing shrinkage, monitoring expired medications, and ensuring proper use of group purchasing organizations (GPOs). Shrinkage is the loss of products as a result of errors, expiration, or theft. Having a good organizational process in place can eliminate much of this shrinkage, and the process can be managed by an advanced technician. Management tasks may include automatic replenishment; periodic auditing of **automated dispensing devices (ADDs)**; ensuring proper storage and shelving; identifying look-alike, sound-alike, and high-risks drugs; and performing organizational quality control measures (Fig. 6.7).

COST

Drug costs will continue to rise, but the use of automated inventory, stock replacement, and order fulfillment systems allows wholesalers to streamline the delivery process and lowers pharmaceutical costs in the supply chain American Society of Health-System Pharmacists [ASHP], (2018). Pharmacies usually enter into contracts with wholesalers known as GPOs, which offer incentives or discounts for drug purchases in most cases. Other benefits for working with GPOs include handling of drug returns, waste management, formulary management, automatic substitution, and automatic delivery or replenishment of automated dispensing systems. All of these practices can be supported by advanced technicians with a knowledge of pharmacology and an understanding of planning and organizational skills.

 Tech Note

On average, patients see their pharmacist 35 times a year, whereas they see their primary care physician about 3 to 4 times a year (Drug Topics, 2019).

STORAGE AND INVENTORY CONTROL

The amount of inventory on hand, essentially, is money sitting on a shelf. The need to overstock certain items, such as antivirals and Tamiflu during flu season, should be incorporated, but during off-seasons, these overstock items should not be stored in excess. If the medication expires or comes close to the expiration date, the loss is taken directly from the pharmacy's bottom line. Manual tracking takes time and does not offer an efficient way to reorder or know what is on hand at any given time. Even the way medications are arranged or stored in ADDs can significantly affect the efficiency of from dispensing.

Management of medication distribution includes centralized and decentralized systems. Decentralized systems use cabinets that contain area- or department-specific medications or floor stock that would typically be required in that area. In this system, there would be a dedicated cabinet with prenatal or OB/GYN supplies on the labor and delivery floor and a cabinet with different types of supplies in the emergency room. This system allows for less duplication and smaller amounts of medications to be stored in the centralized or general pharmacy. The medications and supplies specific to the conditions they are used for are kept only in the areas where they are most appropriate.

In addition, GPOs coordinate automated replenishment through the centralized or decentralized systems. This means that as inventory is depleted, the system knows what needs to be replenished based on a set **periodic automatic replenishment (PAR) level**. Once the amount on hand is set by the facility, the automated system identifies any item that falls under that amount and automatically prepares a delivery for the next day to replenish it.

Although PAR can be accomplished with a decentralized or centralized approach, a decentralized model is often used in hospital systems, in which there are smaller pharmacies, often referred to as *satellites*, located in specific areas, such as the cardiac unit. The specialized pharmacy would have its own stock related to the area it serves, process orders, consult with physicians, and prepare medications on site. The replenishment for this ADD would look different from that at another satellite location.

The centralized model, in contrast, has one main location from which medications are distributed to the patient care areas to be distributed to patients by nurses. The inventory is kept together in one location and distributed from there. This system requires more medications to be kept on hand because all areas must be covered by one location. Although this approach has some advantages for large organizations with many locations, such as lower costs for bulk purchasing, it requires a system of perpetual inventory and a streamlined method for moving medications to areas as they are needed. An advanced technician can support such systems by participating in efforts to improve logistics, storage, and removal of slow-moving medications through ongoing data collection and evaluation.

FLOOR STOCK MANAGEMENT USING AUTOMATION

The maintenance of inventory levels for floor stock, emergency carts, and operating or anesthesia trays can also benefit from automation and verification through RFID or **barcode medication administration (BCMA)** technology (Fig. 6.8). In institutional settings, there are different types of "kits" or "drawers" that include common floor stock or specialty drugs that are replenished for use during procedures. In large hospital systems, these may also include anesthesia or operating room trays, where a set of medications and supplies is made into a kit, and each patient is charged based on which of the items are used. Automated dispensing systems incorporate RFID or BCMA to verify the drugs included in the kit. As another level of verification, an advanced technician can participate in an individual double-check process.

ERROR REDUCTION

As an advanced technician in an inventory support role, being proactive and routinely monitoring supplies and expiration dates or nonmovement from an ADD can help eliminate waste and prevent and reduce errors.

Automated dispensing systems have reporting and auditing capabilities. The visibility of real-time inventory allows for the identification of short-dated medications, usage information, and the current supply in the system. If medications are left unmonitored, the risk of the failure to remove an expired medication increases. Duplication of similar drugs or look-alike drugs in several cabinets can lead to the wrong medication being removed. Knowing what inventory is

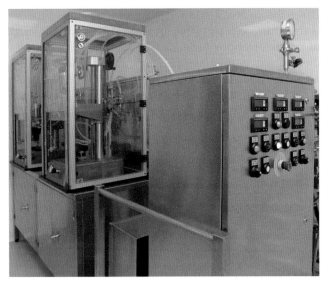

Fig. 6.8 Pharmacy automation. (Copyright © iStock.com/sykono.)

on hand and where it is located can help reduce overages and excess storage of medications in areas where they won't be used. The prevention of adverse events can also be minimized through automation. By using electronic verification methods, the five rights of medication administration can be better managed and improve patient compliance and adherence.

The diversion of controlled substances costs billions of dollars every year and affects many healthcare providers. Automated dispensing systems incorporate a host of reporting features that can be used to track user functions and all functions associated with medications in the system. For example, every time someone signs in, removes a medication, or even opens a drawer in an **automated dispensing cabinet (ADC)**, it is documented with time, date, and the person's identification. Part of the medication-removal process includes the user typing in the beginning inventory of the pocket. If there is a discrepancy between the beginning inventory of the drawer after the removal of a medication, it can be traced back to the users around that time.

SUPPORTING OPTIMAL PATIENT CARE

Another benefit of using automated dispensing technology is the ability to provide safe and efficient patient care. Healthcare personnel who administer medications have access 24/7, and automated replenishing of stock keeps things running smoothly, with no gaps of waiting for a medication that might cause late dosing or administration. Every encounter with the cabinet, patient, or eMAR is electronically available and can be shared or reviewed at any time. For example, if a patient asks for pain medication, the eMAR can be reviewed to determine what medication was given last, at what time, and by whom.

Computerized physician order entry (CPOE) is another important piece of the technology system. In CPOE, the process of entering the physician orders starts the flow of information and closes the loop. After the order is entered electronically, the process is then followed by either BCMA or RFID verification of the medications ordered. The administration of the medication is then verified by reading the patient's armband and that of the care provider who administers the medication. The final stop is a check of the patient's eMAR against the orders entered through the CPOE system.

Case Study

Thinking about the storage and arrangement of medications along with what you learned about workflow in Chapter 5, what would you do in the following situation?

As an advanced technician in the role of inventory technician for a busy hospital, your day starts with an audit of four automated cabinets in the operating room and the recovery room. You finish this task, and upon review of the reports, you find that there are duplications of medications in several cabinets, and in one cabinet, you find several expired medications in some of the pockets. The user reports indicate that the cabinet containing expired medications is only used on weekends, but the stock it contains is almost identical to that of the cabinet just down the hall.

What would be a strategy you could use to decrease shrinkage and the number of expired mediations in these areas?

The best strategy would be to decide if the ADC that contains expired medications is really required for the floor by reviewing the daily information reports provided by suppliers and the tracking technology incorporated in the system. If the cabinet is not being used and the same stock is in other ADCs that are close to the area and can be used conveniently, consider removing the cabinet. In addition, remove any expired medications and any that are close to expiration. The short-dated drugs could be stocked in one of the other department's cabinets if they will be used quickly or returned through the wholesaler.

REMOTE PHARMACY (TELEPHARMACY)

Remote dispensing is another type of technology used in today's pharmacy, especially in rural areas. Many third-party providers include virtual appointment services with primary care providers for patients with acute care needs. Once the medication is prescribed, the next step may include interaction through a video conference in which the pharmacist may counsel the patient and use an ADS to dispense the medication ordered.

In other remote systems, a facility may employ an off-site pharmacist and an on-site advanced technician who prepares medications and then asks for a periodic check (validation) of the work. There are many smaller pharmacies and hospitals that use one remote pharmacist for more than one location and depend on highly qualified technicians to prepare medications for on-site distribution. Such systems may also include a technician who performs remote data entry for pharmacist verification, which is also common in pharmacies today.

COMMON RESPONSIBILITIES FOR ADVANCED TECHNICIANS WORKING WITH TECHNOLOGY OR AUTOMATED DISPENSING SYSTEMS

Advanced technicians can perform operational functions to support the automated dispensing systems and technology used by the pharmacy. For example, a pharmacy-automation specialist or a pharmacy ADC quality coordinator may perform the following common duties (ASHP, 2017):

- Performing maintenance and new build-outs for systems
- Facilitating start-ups, installations, and expansions as needed
- Managing users (e.g., activating and deactivating passwords)

- Making formulary changes, such as adjusting PAR levels and completing removals as a result of short dates or outdates
- Training other staff
- Auditing and reporting on system functions and efficiency
- Quality control, including error reduction and reporting of adverse effects
- Auditing for discrepancies (user removals and inventory)

Supporting roles for advanced technicians who work with technology and automated dispensing systems are very important in the operations of today's pharmacy. These can also include working in a support role by performing searches of the databases of prescription-monitoring programs. These are state-run programs that collect data on controlled drug prescriptions as part of an effort to prevent drug addiction and abuse. The reporting capabilities of advanced dispensing systems allow useful information to be reviewed and distributed by the organizations using them and by regulatory agencies. Common roles in this area include the pharmacy loss prevention specialist, who performs the following functions (ASHP, 2017):

- Conducting audits for controlled substances (orders, invoices, shipments, and logs)
- Updating and informing other staff regarding local, state, and federal laws
- Conducting staff training
- Investigating any fraudulent or suspicious activity
- Ensuring compliance with regulations for cash-handling activities
- Working with internal leadership to promote awareness and make recommendations for process improvements

Another area involving technology is the support role in performing data analysis for streamlining information systems and communication. For technicians interested in the technology related to pharmacy-related equipment, such as smart pumps, ADCs, and eMARs, there are also informatics technician positions.

For technicians who wish to advance in the areas of technology or informatics (information systems), there are many opportunities in today's pharmacy. Organizations are looking for technologically savvy and energetic technicians with a background in pharmacology, organizational skills, and an understanding of processes.

Today's lean, quality-driven climate demands that pharmacies increase efficiency and use the talents available while providing the highest-quality patient care.

REVIEW QUESTIONS

1. Which of the following is NOT one of the five rights of medication administration?
   a. Right dose
   b. Right time
   c. Right route
   d. Right package

2. Which of the following tracking methods uses radio waves to transmit data?
   a. BCMA
   b. RFID
   c. NDC
   d. None of the above

3. Which of the following identification methods must use a scanner to read the codes?
   a. RFID
   b. NDC
   c. CPOE
   d. BCMA

4. Which of the following is the process of entering physician orders into a database electronically?
   a. CPOE
   b. RFID
   c. BCMA
   d. NDC

5. Which of the following is the identification method that uses 10 digits to represent the labeler, product, and packaging?
   a. NDC
   b. RFID
   c. GPO
   d. Barcode

6. Which is the best method of recording the administration of a patient's medication?
   a. Enter it in the eMAR once it has been given.
   b. Print it in the chart right after giving it.
   c. Communicate it through a telephone call right after giving it.
   d. Leave a detailed note for the next shift.

7. All of the following are methods by which an ADD tracks the personnel who use it EXCEPT:
   a. Recording of every entry
   b. Use of barcode scanner
   c. Running reports
   d. CPOE entry

8. What term is used to identify the amount of a medication that is set to be kept on hand?
   a. BCMA
   b. CPOE
   c. ACD
   d. PAR

9. Which of the following is an example of an open-ended question?
   a. Is your name Charles?
   b. Is your birthday in May?
   c. What is your address?
   d. All of the above

10. Which term describes the pharmacy system that uses satellite pharmacies?
    a. Decentralized
    b. Centralized
    c. Inpatient
    d. Outpatient

CRITICAL THINKING QUESTIONS

1. As a pharmacy informatics technician in a busy hospital, you are tasked with streamlining the communication between automated systems and those tracking other equipment, such as smart pumps. There have been some delays in patients receiving their treatments and disconnects in the relaying of information from one system to another. What would you include in a plan to address the issues?
2. Discuss the flow of the different technologies involved from the point of a physician ordering a medication to the final check of its administration.

REFERENCES

ASHP, (2017). Advanced Pharmacy Technician Roles. Retrieved July 21, 2020 from https://www.ashp.org/Pharmacy-Technician/About-Pharmacy-Technicians/Advanced-Pharmacy-Technician-Roles?loginreturnUrl=SSOCheckOnly.

American Society of Health-System Pharmacists. (2018). ASHP guidelines on medication cost management strategies for hospitals and health systems. *Am J Health-Syst Pharm, 65,* 1368–1384.

Brewin, B. (2004). FDA Backs RFID Tags to Track Prescription Drugs. Retrieved July 22, 2020 from https://www.computerworld.com/article/2575009/fda-backs-rfid-tags-to-track-prescription-drugs.html.

Drug Topics. The Future of Pharmacy Automation. Retrieved October 30, 2019 from https://drugtopics.com/automation/future-pharmacy-automation/page/0/3.

Advanced Clinical Skills in Community and Institutional Settings

Learning Objectives

1. Discuss how the evolution of pharmacy practice provides expanded opportunities for technicians in advanced clinical roles.
2. List some of today's clinical practices where pharmacy participates to support value-based care and the patient-centered model.
3. Identify some of the opportunities available for the advanced clinical pharmacy technician.
4. List common skills required of advanced clinical technicians in both community and institutional pharmacy settings.

Key Terms

Pharmacogenetics The relationship of how one's genes react to different medications; often used interchangeably with *pharmacogenomics*.

Pharmacokinetics The study of the movement of drugs throughout the body.

Protocol A series of guidelines for a patient to follow that are based on a series of visits or screenings used to achieve a health-related goal.

INTRODUCTION

Traditionally, technicians have served in a behind-the-scenes or supporting role when it came to clinical interaction with customers or patients. Although they processed payments, handed out or delivered medication, and performed data entry, the counseling or delivery of information was provided by a pharmacist. With the evolution of pharmacies providing a host of clinical pharmacy services, the advanced technician often serves in the front or has direct patient contact. The patient-centered approach must include a support model that aligns each team member toward a common goal of achieving a patient's therapeutic outcomes, which goes far beyond just dispensing medication. Pharmacists have transitioned their practice to work directly with patients and other care providers to participate in the value-based system. This requires them to delegate the technical duties to competent staff, which often includes experienced or advanced technicians (Fig. 7.1). This provides opportunities for clinical services to be performed by advanced technicians who wish to be more directly involved with the patient. Organizations must evaluate the impact of the services and coordinate the budgets and staffing requirements in today's fast-paced environment. The use of clinically oriented technicians to provide direct clinical support is one of the best ways to do this.

EVOLUTION OF CLINICAL SERVICES PROVIDED BY TODAY'S PHARMACY

There are many changes in the role that pharmacy plays in today's patient care compared with the past. Although the pharmacist is still responsible for all decisions requiring clinical judgment, the gathering of data, evaluation and recording of processes, and triaging of patients can be performed by advanced technicians with the proper training. Optimizing the skills and knowledge of advanced technicians in clinical roles provides cost-saving and time-saving benefits to an organization.

New clinical services offered by today's pharmacy include direct interaction with the patient in almost a primary care role. Functioning as a clinic, the pharmacy provides convenient patient care for common ailments, offers vaccinations, performs physicals and health screenings, and more. To be able to devote the time needed for patients and participate directly with other care providers on the patient's behalf, pharmacists must have confidence in their technicians. As an integral part of the healthcare team, technicians serving in advanced roles can support and assist in providing the highest-quality and safest care for a patient.

Providing services as a community clinic is a significant part of modern pharmacy practice today. Many third-party insurance providers require employees to maintain a point-value system that monitors

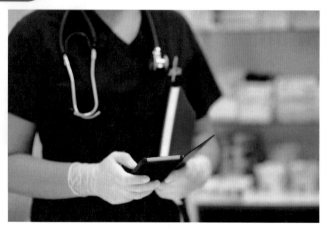

Fig. 7.1 Clinical technician using technology to research medications. (Copyright © iStock.com/SbytovaMN.)

lifestyle and preventive testing or screenings as part of a wellness-promotion approach. As part of this approach, pharmacy technicians can be trained to perform point-of-care testing (POCT) under a pharmacist's supervision. Expanded clinical services can include demonstration techniques for blood glucose meters and inhalers; fittings for Jobst stockings or special shoes or inserts for diabetics; and discussion of over-the-counter tests, such as pregnancy and drug tests. Expanded clinical services also involve billing and coding for services, such as Medicare coding. The durable medical equipment Medicare coding category includes walkers, crutches, wheelchairs, oxygen, and other items many community pharmacies provide.

POINT-OF-CARE TESTING

POCT includes common diagnostic tests that can aid in the early detection of conditions or diseases and acute conditions such as strep or flu. In 1988, the United States congress passed the Clinical Laboratory Improvement Amendments (CLIA) to regulate all facilities that perform laboratory testing. Regardless of whether the lab is large or small, the goal of CLIA was to ensure the same test would yield the same results regardless of where it is performed or by whom. CLIA accomplishes this through rigid quality control and certification standards, including onsite surveys. The Centers for Medicare and Medicaid Services (CMS) inspects and certifies laboratories, while the Food and Drug Administration (FDA) regulates all laboratory tests performed on humans. The FDA classifies laboratory tests by complexity. Certain tests require years of training and advanced scientific knowledge to perform, and errors in the testing process will occur without extensive laboratory expertise. Other laboratory tests are categorized as moderately complex—these do not require the highest levels of training to perform, but do require the skills of a laboratory professional. Still others the FDA has determined have a low risk of erroneous results; these are called *waived* tests, because they can be performed at sites without the most

rigorous CLIA requirements. The FDA has waived many tests that can be provided in today's modern pharmacy, however, the pharmacy must be certified through CLIA in order to bill Medicaid or Medicare for these tests. In some cases, when a test result is positive, some states allow related prescribing rights for medications such as antibiotics or antivirals.

Tech Note

Did you know that CVS has over 1100 Minute Clinics in 33 states operated by healthcare professionals, including physicians, nurses, pharmacists, and technicians? To date, there have been over 37 million patient visits recorded. See https://www.cvs.com/minuteclinic for more information.

A complete list of waived tests can be found at https://www.cms.gov/Regulations-and-Guidance/Legislation/CLIA/Downloads/waivetbl.pdf. Current Procedural Terminology (CPT) codes are 5-digit numbers used to identify and bill services such as surgery or medicine. Common tests performed in pharmacies today include the following:

- Strep throat—swab to determine the presence of streptococcus bacteria
- Influenza tests
- Lipid profiles—tests for cholesterol, triglycerides, or high-density lipoprotein (HDL) in whole blood
- Pregnancy and ovulation tests
- Fecal occult blood (Hemoccult) or colorectal screening—tests for blood in feces
- Blood glucose—tests for amount of glucose in blood (diabetes)
- Urinalysis—can tests for illicit drugs, glucose, blood, ketones, urinary tract infection (UTI), or kidney function
- Gastroccult—tests for pH in gastric juices (acid–base balance); used in determining gastroesophageal reflux disease (GERD)
- Male fertility (sperm count)
- A1C tests—measure concentration of hemoglobin A1C; used in long-term care of patients with diabetes
- Vaginal pH detection tests
- Thyroid tests—determine function of thyroid; used in diagnosing hypothyroidism
- Blood platelets or clotting tests—used for patients on warfarin (Coumadin) or heparin; also can be used in diagnosing vitamin K deficiencies

It should be noted that a waived test does not mean it is foolproof, or that errors would not cause life-changing or even fatal effects. For example, a false positive on a drug test could cost someone their job; an inaccurate blood glucose result could send a patient into a diabetic crisis; an erroneous clotting test would cause a patient to take the wrong dose of anticoagulant, potentially resulting in a stroke, heart attack, or internal bleeding. For these reasons the trained pharmacy technician should perform all testing with professionalism and diligence, following all quality control procedures.

COUNSELING PROGRAMS

In addition to POCT, pharmacies are also providing counseling services, such as smoking cessation and alcohol awareness. Several states allow pharmacists to prescribe smoking cessation aids. A new Medicare Part B regulation allows for two smoking cessation counseling services each year for those who are using tobacco. In addition, some over-the-counter (OTC) nicotine replacement aids are now covered by Medicaid. The pharmacist serves as a liaison between the patient's primary care provider and continues the treatment toward a healthier lifestyle and monitoring of progression through a cessation program.

The advanced clinical technician can provide support by recording or tracking progress; maintaining current test results, such as A1C; and documenting information required in a medication management plan.

Advanced technicians can use their previous experience, organizational skills, and critical thinking to evaluate and assist in tracking results and collaborating with other team members if further evaluation is needed. Through a screening process, if values are noted as abnormal, the technician can alert the pharmacist and help organize consultations if needed. Scheduling and notifying the patient of an upcoming session are important duties that allow pharmacists to use their expertise and training during the actual patient consult. Billing for the actual consult time is limited by most third-party providers, and providing a history and results from tests before the consult allows the pharmacist to review the patient's record prior to a visit.

IMMUNIZATION PROGRAMS

Many pharmacies now administer vaccines or immunizations, such as the influenza, shingles, Tdap, and both adult pneumococcal vaccines (Fig. 7.2). This is now very common, and third-party providers can be billed for these vaccinations and immunizations. The advanced technician can play an important role in this service. For example, if the patient's coverage falls under the medical benefit category, the advanced technician will know how to successfully and efficiently submit the claim, ensuring the pharmacy will receive payment for services. The process includes different computer relays for messaging along with network credentialing. Technicians can enter prescriptions in the database, prepare syringes, and record storage information. In addition, any patient leaflets or information can be printed or completed by the technician if required by a third party for reimbursement. Technicians serving in a more advanced role can schedule patients and collect the patient's medical history, such as previous vaccines, allergies, or reactions. In Idaho, technicians who complete a required training program can administer vaccines under state regulations.

Managing clinical projects, such as an outcome tracking program, and evaluating existing ones can assist the organization in determining which screening and prevention methods are working. Identifying payers, setting up scheduled visits, and maintaining the proper level of inventory to accommodate the time of year during which the vaccine should be stocked are also key aspects of a successful immunization program. For example, the flu season often results in backorders of vaccines, and many community pharmacies schedule special days each month for vaccinations. If the stock level is not appropriate for the days advertised, it can cause scheduling issues and a loss of profit to the store. Thinking ahead and being prepared can be significant assets in vaccination programs (Fig. 7.3).

 Tech Note

Forty-eight states, the District of Columbia, and Puerto Rico allow pharmacists to administer vaccines, and Idaho currently allows properly trained technicians to administer vaccines.

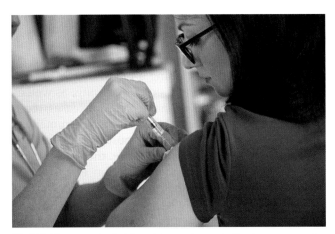

Fig. 7.2 Pharmacy technician giving an immunization in a community pharmacy clinic setting. (Copyright © iStock.com/fstop123.)

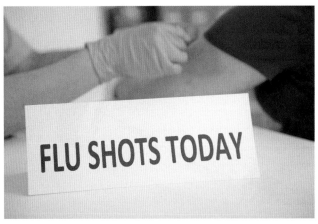

Fig. 7.3 Flu shots. (Copyright © iStock.com/fstop123.)

LONG-ACTING MEDICATION PROGRAMS

In some states, pharmacists are allowed to administer long-acting drugs, such as vitamin B_{12} monthly injections or a one-time methotrexate injection used in ectopic pregnancies. In addition, some antipsychotic agents, such as Once a month Haldol deconoate injections for the treatment of schizophrenia, can be administered by pharmacists. This medication can be administered intramuscularly, either every 14 or 28 days (Fig. 7.4). Long-acting medication programs usually involve a partnership with another care provider, such as a mental health provider in the case of decanoate or a women's clinic for methotrexate.

An advanced clinical technician can support this service by performing clinical administrative duties, such as tracking the injections, recording any adverse reactions, and coordinating with other providers to set up appointments. Maintenance of the injection schedule is extremely important because these medications are released over a specific number of days, and being late can cause significant side effects, especially for patients with schizophrenia, who are often not high functioning and need additional attention to stay on track with medications and maintain adherence to the regimen they are prescribed. As the support technician, helping to keep the patient informed and other care providers involved is essential to the overall health and wellness of the patient.

CONTRACEPTIVE PRESCRIBING PROGRAM

Currently, several states allow pharmacists to prescribe hormonal contraceptives (Fig. 7.5). In an effort to reduce the unintended pregnancy rate, there is a nationwide push to work toward awareness and to provide contraceptives for underprivileged or uninformed populations. These medications are available at little or low cost from several online companies and through Medicaid, and some third-party providers either offer them or, in some cases, pay a reimbursement fee for a pharmacist to prescribe them. This reimbursement fee may include a 30- to 45-minute consultation and dispensing of the contraceptive chosen. Advanced clinical

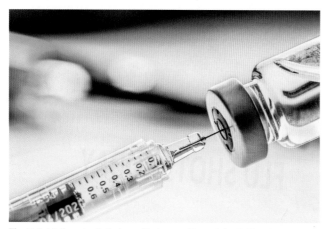

Fig. 7.4 Vial contents being withdrawn. (Copyright © iStock.com/MarianVejcik.)

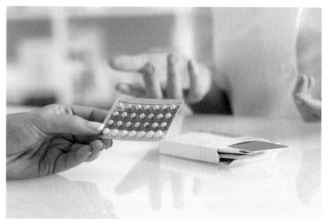

Fig. 7.5 Pharmacist discussing a contraceptive choice. (Copyright © iStock.com/AntonioGuillem.)

technicians can provide support for such programs, including documenting and screening patients, recording medical and medication histories, setting up appointments, and working directly with other primary care providers. Providing basic information and collecting the correct payment information for the pharmacist prior to a consultation or dispensing of medication are cost efficient and beneficial to the organization.

 Tech Note

Contraceptives can be prescribed by pharmacists in California, Colorado, Hawaii, New Mexico, Oregon, Tennessee, and Washington.

PHARMACOGENETIC TESTING PROGRAMS

As advances in medications and knowledge of diseases and conditions increase, new treatments and diagnostic efforts emerge. **Pharmacogenetics** is how a person's genes react to medications. For example, if a person metabolizes medication slower than another, the dose may need to be different from that for someone who metabolizes it faster to achieve the same effect. One example of a class of drugs that may be included in pharmacogenetic testing programs is psychiatric drugs.

Early detection and genetic predisposition information can give the pharmacist and provider vital information prior to prescribing a medication (Fig. 7.6). This saves a lot of trial and error in dosing, as well as the time it takes to make changes; in some cases, it can prevent the loss of revenue that occurs when medications have to be changed and disposed of. Every time there is a dose or medication change, there is a higher risk of adverse effects and medication errors, along with additional costs to the pharmacy for medications that have to be disposed of.

With the value-based approach also comes the need to prevent diseases years ahead of detection or before clues are seen. For example, in many cases, monitoring

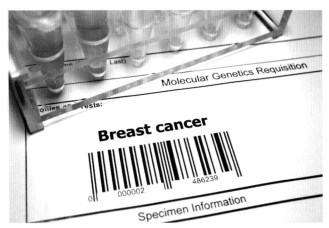

Fig. 7.6 DNA testing of genes for breast cancer. (Copyright © iStock. com/Hailshadow.)

and controlling blood pressure or glucose levels can prevent major events or diseases, such as heart attacks and diabetes, from occurring. Pharmacists' knowledge of **pharmacokinetics**, drug transport, and metabolism can also help to optimize patients' response to medications. This clinical information is reviewed by the pharmacist, and recommendations for dosing can be shared with the primary care physician.

Additionally, preparing a medication management plan for each individual is a way to create a patient-specific plan with outcomes based on testing, adherence to medication regimens, and even healthy lifestyles. Advanced clinical technicians can support such programs through direct clinical services support, such as organizing clinical data or identifying values that are considered to be outside the normal range. In addition, the patient's history (medication and health) information must be recorded and updated regularly for review by the pharmacist at any given time.

Case Study

You are working in an advanced role as an emergency department liaison who collects medication histories when patients are moved to the floor, transferred to another facility, or discharged home. The patient's handwritten list of medications and the verbal list from the family are not matching up. The patient and family didn't bring bottles for confirmation, and the patient is being transferred to a long-term facility. What would be the best way to ensure the correct medications are recorded? Once you have the list, what would you do with this information?

Ask where the patient's prescriptions are being filled (e.g., drugstore) and call that store. If there is more than one, call all of them. Once the correct list is obtained, it should be entered in the appropriate facility records and shared with the pharmacist. Note any duplications, late or early refills, or outstanding medications ordered but not obtained for the pharmacist to review prior to counseling the patient.

OPPORTUNITIES FOR ADVANCED CLINICAL TECHNICIANS IN COMMUNITY AND INSTITUTIONAL SETTINGS

Providing clinical services in the community setting is very common today. Large chains such as CVS and Walgreens and companies like Amazon have begun to pay for training for healthcare positions or careers for their employees through partnerships with educational institutions. Such programs are costly, but the benefits of having a trained workforce include increased patient safety and, in the long run, a more efficient way to provide quality care to patients and customers. The range of responsibilities is growing and will continue to expand.

Some of the common community services being offered today by these organizations include facilities or clinics such as the following:
- Home infusion (compounding) centers
- Mail-order centers or triage centers for pharmacist-administered services
- Long-term care centers
- Call centers
- Acute or on-site clinics

SKILLS REQUIRED OF THE ADVANCED CLINICAL PHARMACY TECHNICIAN

Large corporate settings often incorporate advanced technicians. Such companies seek advanced technicians who have special skill sets to perform a host of clinical services, such as the following:
- Accepting oral orders
- Transferring prescriptions
- Remote prescription processing or mail-order interpretation
- Point of care testing
- Vaccine administration documentation
- Sterile and nonsterile compounding

The skills required for advanced clinical roles in these settings must include excellent interpersonal and personal skills. This allows the advanced technician to interact appropriately with other healthcare providers and patients and communicate in a professional manner (Fig. 7.7). Assisting with medication reconciliation or medication management requires advanced knowledge of pharmacology and anatomy. The information collected must be correct, including spelling, description, and proper use of grammar. Knowledge of Microsoft programs, such as Excel and Word, is necessary to complete most forms, so computer and typing skills are a must.

Good math skills are also required because clinical technicians often interpret laboratory test results and participate in dispensing using advanced technology. This may include reviewing data, computing statistics, or performing tracking of errors through audits. Advanced technicians may be involved in managing clinical projects through protocol-based screening

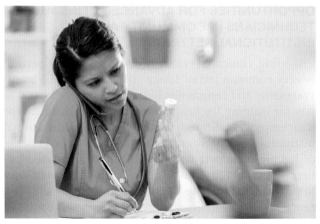

Fig. 7.7 Pharmacy technician talking to another healthcare provider about medications. (Copyright © iStock.com/SDI-Productions .)

or outcome tracking. A **protocol** is a series of rules or parameters that would be set for a patient to meet to achieve a certain outcome. For example, it could involve screenings that are scored to determine a predetermined level of performance.

The advanced technician is also invaluable in roles involving compounding. The actual preparation of intravenous (IV) sterile and nonsterile preparations is performed by the technician so that the pharmacist can concentrate on dosing regimens and patient response to therapy. The technician's role also includes interpretation of orders, calculations for preparation, and knowledge of US Pharmacopeia (USP) guidelines (see discussion in Chapter 10).

Advanced technicians must have a good understanding of pharmacology, usual dosing, laws and regulations, and disease processes because several states allow certified technicians to be more directly involved in accepting orders or prescriptions. For example:

- Iowa—Certified pharmacy technicians (CPhTs) can accept new orders and refill authorizations from prescribers or authorized persons.
- Idaho—CPhTs can transfer orders for the purpose of refilling through fax, electronic, or verbal communications from a prescriber or authorized person.
- Ohio—CPhTs can accept new orders that are written, faxed, or sent electronically. Orders for noncontrolled drugs from a prescriber or an authorized person can be accepted verbally.

Advanced technicians' participation in more clinical roles allows for pharmacists to engage in the evolving role toward patient care provider. Triaging patients to aid pharmacists in deciding which services to provide and when, serving as discharge or admission advocates, and recording and tracking medication histories are also important because these clinical functions support today's patient-centered model. At today's pharmacies, all professionals work together as a team to provide patients with affordable, high-quality services.

REVIEW QUESTIONS

1. Which of the following states allows pharmacy technicians to legally administer immunizations?
   a. Ohio
   b. Indiana
   c. Iowa
   d. Idaho
2. All of the following states allow technicians to accept verbal orders EXCEPT:
   a. Iowa
   b. Indiana
   c. Ohio
   d. Idaho
3. Which of the following point-of-care tests could be used to diagnose GERD?
   a. A1C
   b. Hemoccult
   c. Urinalysis
   d. Gastroccult
4. Which of the following states allows pharmacists to legally prescribe contraceptives?
   a. Colorado
   b. Georgia
   c. Kentucky
   d. Utah
5. Which of the following point-of-care tests would be most appropriate to use for the long-term care of a patient with diabetes?
   a. A1C
   b. Urinalysis
   c. Tuberculosis
   d. Gastroccult
6. How many states currently allow pharmacists to prescribe contraceptives?
   a. Seven
   b. Six
   c. Five
   d. Four
7. Which is the study of the way a person's genes react to medications?
   a. Physiology
   b. Pharmacokinetics
   c. Pharmacogenetics
   d. Pharmacology
8. If a patient is treated for high blood pressure through a series of scheduled visits and periodic screenings, what would this be called?
   a. Pharmacogenetics
   b. Pharmacology
   c. Pharmacokinetics
   d. Protocol

9. Which of the following long-acting medications is given every 14 to 28 days for the treatment of schizophrenia?
   a. Vitamin B$_{12}$
   b. Methotrexate
   c. Haldol decanoate
   d. None of the above

10. Which of the following long-acting injections can be given for an ectopic pregnancy?
   a. Vitamin B$_{12}$
   b. Methotrexate
   c. Haldol
   d. None of the above

11. Which of the following medications is given for the treatment of anemia?
   a. Vitamin B$_{12}$
   b. Methotrexate
   c. Haldol
   d. None of the above

CRITICAL THINKING QUESTIONS

1. Describe how the value-based approach can help prevent future hospitalizations or even life-threatening events.

2. Describe how an advanced clinical technician could assist a pharmacist in an immunization clinic.

REFERENCES

CMS.gov. Tests Granted Waive Status Under CLIA. Retrieved November 7, 2019 from https://www.cms.gov/Regulations-and-Guidance/Legislation/CLIA/Downloads/waivetbl.pdf.

CMS.gov. Clinical Laboratory Improvement Amendments. Retrieved November 7, 2019 from https://www.cms.gov/Regulations-and-Guidance/Legislation/CLIA/index.html.

Krizner, K. Training Technicians for More Responsibility. Retrieved November 11, 2019 from https://www.drugtopics.com/health-system-news/training-technicians-more-responsibility/page/0/1.

Tzipora Lieder. Latest Six New Clinical Services for Pharmacist. Retrieved November 9, 2019 from https://www.drugtopics.com/latest/six-new-clinical-services-pharmacists/page/0/1?utm_source=bibblio_recommendation.

8 Patient Medication Compliance and Monitoring

Learning Objectives

1. Define *medication adherence* and explain its importance in a patient's overall health and in our healthcare system model today.
2. Discuss common types of medication nonadherence and how the roles of advanced technicians can assist in the process of improvement.
3. Discuss barriers to medication adherence and strategies for improvement.
4. Discuss the role of medication reconciliation and the advanced technician's role in the process.

Key Terms

Acute condition An abrupt onset of a disease or condition.

Chronic condition A condition that persists for longer than 3 months and is ongoing.

Medication reconciliation Process of creating the most accurate list of medications used in medication adherence programs.

Value-based care System based on accountability; payments for services are based on outcomes rather than volume.

INTRODUCTION

Medication adherence, sometimes referred to as *patient compliance*, includes several factors. In general, it refers to the extent to which patients take their prescribed medication. It's a collaboration between a healthcare provider and the patient to follow a set of instructions meant to improve the patient's health (Fig. 8.1). This also includes adherence to a provider's recommendations for behavior, lifestyle, or treatments designed to improve or prevent a worsening of the disease or condition. Patients are said to be adherent to therapy if they take their prescribed medication at least 80% of the time (Kadia & Schroeder, 2015).

THE IMPORTANCE OF MEDICATION ADHERENCE

Clearly, failing to take medication as prescribed can have adverse consequences for the patient's health. If the patient is not taking medications, then the drugs are not producing the desired effects on the body. Furthermore, the provider is making decisions about the patient's treatment under the assumption that the patient is taking medications as ordered. Without seeing the expected results, the provider may switch treatments or add other medications unnecessarily, causing additional health problems.

Poor adherence not only affects the individual patient but also the overall healthcare system (Fig. 8.2). As discussed earlier (Chapter 5), the current model of **value-based care** focuses on the predetermined outcomes for the patient rather than the successful completion of a series of tests or clinical appointments. This is accomplished by monitoring adherence to healthy lifestyle guidelines and medication regimens and supporting the patient continuously. Establishing a series of ongoing efforts to improve and prevent events related to a patient's chronic condition or disease can prevent the worsening of the disease or condition.

The cost to the country's healthcare system becomes quite evident with repeated hospital stays for preventable events, such as heart attacks resulting from nonadherence to medication, lack of monitoring of blood pressure, or poor lifestyle choices. Advanced technicians' current direct engagement with patients in a variety of settings provides an important link between the patient and the provider or pharmacist. This link has proven to be invaluable in the team approach to today's value-based system.

In today's competitive healthcare environment, pharmacies must provide the highest-quality services, and they rely on payment from results-oriented systems, such as bonus payment incentives. Pharmacies must focus on improving patient care and educating providers because the performance of medication adherence is reflected in reimbursement.

The Centers for Medicare and Medicaid Services (CMS) is a federal agency within the US Department of Health and Human Services (HHS). This organization has created the Star rating system, which provides payments or reimbursement to providers based on a

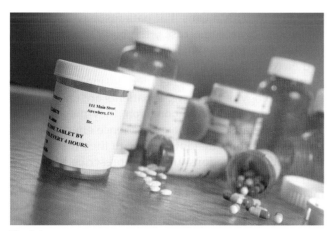

Fig. 8.1 Multiple medications for one patient. (Copyright © iStock/fstop123.)

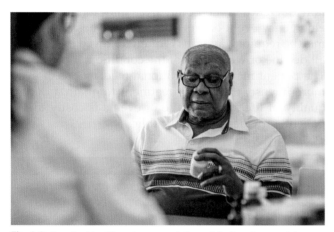

Fig. 8.2 A patient looking at a prescription while the pharmacist explains the importance of adherence. (Copyright @ iStock/FatCamera.)

scoring system. Several of these ratings are tied directly to patient medication adherence and the impacts on patients' overall health. These include the following:

- Improvement—rating of 5
- Outcomes—rating of 3
- Intermediate outcomes—rating of 3
- Patient experience—1.5
- Access—rating of 1.5
- Process—rating of 1

Bonuses are awarded to insurers that offer private coverage to Medicare beneficiaries that receive ratings of 4 or higher. These can be in the form of direct bonus payments or rebates.

Diseases such as diabetes and hypertension can be prevented or managed with proper medication adherence, and this also reduces costs to the system. Nonadherence to medication can result in a waste of medication, the progression of a disease or condition, a lower quality of life, and repeated hospital visits. All of these costs affect each of us and take a huge toll on the healthcare system and the public. Keeping the patient well is the best for all parties involved. In addition to the far-reaching economic effects, medication

nonadherence is also related to antibiotic resistance and research regarding the value of many medications and the target conditions they relate to. In order to judge the true results of medication effects, the drug must be taken properly as prescribed. Future development depends on results and the outcomes achieved by large groups of patients. To make decisions on new medications, companies depend on accurate results derived from patients taking the medication as it was designed.

Pharmacies are currently scored on the following areas:

- Management of chronic conditions through medication adherence
- Medication safety, especially in high-risk populations (e.g., elderly patients)
- Completion of medication therapy management (MTM) program documentation

  Ways to boost these ratings include the following:
- Counseling patients
- Watching for drug interactions or duplications
- Offering medication-synchronizing services
- Communicating with other providers regularly
- Maintaining accurate electronic records

Advanced technicians can play a significant role in the pharmacy's ability to raise Star ratings by participating in these endeavors.

TYPES OF MEDICATION NONADHERENCE

There are many reasons patients do not adhere to medication instructions, as discussed later in this chapter. Advanced technicians can play a significant role in facilitating adherence if they have a proper understanding and awareness of how to identify the types of nonadherence.

 Tech Note

Medication nonadherence results in over 125,000 deaths and $290 billion in costs each year in the United States (Benjamin, 2012).

NONFULFILLMENT ADHERENCE

In this instance, the provider orders a prescription and the patient never fills it. Patients are often resistant to following up with a provider's instructions for medications. They will initially go to an appointment because of an acute or chronic condition, such as pain or something that has impeded their normal activity. Once this is completed, they do not follow through with the provider's treatment plan, which could include medication. They may have gotten an answer regarding the reason they initially went to see the provider, and that's enough. In other cases, the treatment could cost more than they can afford, take time they don't think they have, or interfere with what they consider their normal daily routine. They may think

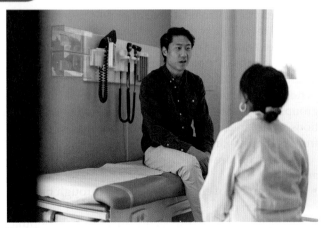

Fig. 8.3 Patient discussing medications with his provider. (Copyright @ iStock/FatCamera.)

that because they have a diagnosis, they can find an over-the-counter, easier, and cheaper alternative route that will do the same job as the prescription they don't want to get filled (Fig. 8.3).

NONPERSISTENCE ADHERENCE

If patients do decide to get their prescription filled, they may take it at first but not complete the recommended course. This is especially an issue with antibiotics. Once patients feel better, they often just stop taking the medication. Sometimes this is intentional, and sometimes it is not. If there is no ongoing engagement between the pharmacy and a provider to encourage adherence, patients may not complete the full course of medication. Nonpersistence adherence can be related to costs as well if the patient does not see the value of continuing to get refills and taking the medication, especially in cases of controlling chronic conditions or disease progression.

The patient must be educated by the pharmacy and providers in how noncontrolled management of many diseases, such as diabetes or blood pressure, can result in emergencies or life-threatening events. Patients may feel fine and not realize that continued adherence to medication is maintaining their quality of life.

This type of nonadherence can also be related to improper instructions given initially, such as inhaler directions. If patients pick up the prescription and are not directed as to how to administer the doses, they may feel the medication is not improving their breathing and stop using the inhaler. Again, this is why it is so important to ensure that patients understand what they are taking the medication for and when to take or administer it.

NONCONFORMING ADHERENCE

Patients often take their medications based on a schedule that aligns with their current lifestyle rather than what is prescribed. This leads to skipping doses, taking doses too close together, or getting higher or lower doses that may not metabolize as the medication is

designed to. This means that patients may not get the full doses, or in some cases, the body's systems will eliminate the excess when doses are taken too close together. Medications are formulated to achieve the best results, which includes scheduled dosing based on the pharmacology of the drug. If patients are taking medication to treat an **acute condition**, they may be more adherent because they may experience effects such as pain or symptoms that interfere with their normal routine. If the medications are being prescribed to maintain or treat a **chronic condition**, such as diabetes, they may be apt to forget to take their medications because there are no apparent signs of discomfort or reasons to adjust their lifestyle. Therefore, existing conditions, such as diabetes and chronic pulmonary obstructive disease (COPD), are harder to manage because patients don't experience symptoms or see the results of nonadherence in their daily lives until a trauma or an emergency event occurs. By this time, hospitalization may be required, and this is often followed by an overall decline or worsening of the condition, if not death. The patient may need additional medications or even more intense, expensive treatment to attain a decent quality of life. This cascade of events is costly to the patient, providers, and the public.

 Tech Note

Did you know that high blood pressure is also known as the "silent killer," and only about half of adults between the ages of 35 and 64 have it under control? It usually has no symptoms until after it has done significant damage to the heart (American Heart Association, 2020).

BARRIERS TO MEDICATION ADHERENCE

Treating most conditions or diseases today involves a comprehensive team approach that includes the involvement of several healthcare providers. The complexity of managing lifestyle, medication regimens, and supportive treatments or routine testing takes time from busy work schedules and requires organization. Patients often see their regular provider as well as specialists and keep track of their own care and medication adherence plan. For children or the elderly, this responsibility falls to an adult caregiver. With so many different elements and people involved, it is easy to see how patients can become confused and unable to manage their medications without a supportive system to provide assistance.

MISCOMMUNICATION WITH PROVIDERS

Starting with the provider, the importance of good communication cannot be underestimated. It is a key element of the patient-centered care approach because all treatment plans must include patients in their own care. The patient must understand instructions for medications, the importance of treatment plans, and the importance of adherence to any lifestyle or supportive treatments that are ordered.

Some studies report that 40% to 60% of patients were unable to relay what the provider expected of them a mere 10 minutes after the information was provided (Jimmy & Jose, 2011), which could have a significant effect in the basic stages of building a successful plan for the patient to manage diseases or conditions. In some cases, it may result from a lack of good communication between the caregiver and patient. This could be attributable to language barriers, socioeconomic differences, or an apathetic attitude of the provider. Patients may have low literacy and may not have a clear understanding of the consequences of missing medication doses, or they may be unable to understand or read instructions, which can lead to poor management of their medication.

FEAR OF ADVERSE EFFECTS OF THE DRUGS

Some patients may not ever start a medication because of a fear of the adverse effects, such as blurred vision, increased appetite, or drowsiness, and others may stop taking medications as soon as the adverse effects begin. It is important that patients are informed of the time it will take to see a positive effect and also understand that in many cases, the adverse effects will subside, and given enough time, they will feel better once the drug builds in their system. This is often the case for mental health medications, for example. Many of the drugs used to treat schizophrenia or depression take 6 weeks or longer to show full effects, but the adverse effects may present much sooner than this. With adverse effects being prominent, patients may focus only on these and not the long-term benefits of managing the disease.

NOT CONVINCED OF THE NEED FOR THE TREATMENT OR MEDICATIONS

Many patients who have chronic diseases, such as hypertension, see their providers regularly and adhere to routine tests or treatments, such as prothrombin time (PT)/international normalized ratio (INR) for blood clotting, A1C for diabetes, or thyroid function, that can indicate ongoing diseases or conditions. However, there are some who are not convinced that following recommendations for the times in between visits is just as important as attending the periodic appointments. This is because they are not motivated or informed enough to understand that periodic testing and visits are designed to monitor what they do daily that determines their quality of life. For example, they may receive lab values for cholesterol and triglycerides that are in line with the previous readings (slightly elevated) but are told their weight has increased. Without a clear understanding that obesity can greatly affect their heart function and raise these values later in life, they continue the same behaviors and gain more weight. Unless an event occurs, they just see the medications prescribed as something they

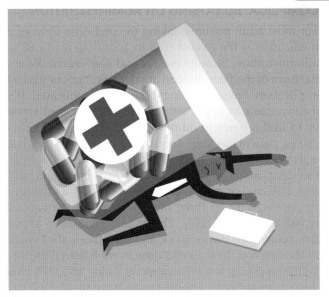

Fig. 8.4 Overwhelming costs of medications. (Copyright @ iStock/sorbetto.)

should do because the provider said to. Over time, they may become complacent and stop taking their medication because they feel fine.

COST AND ACCESS

The cost of medication is one of the biggest factors in medication nonadherence (Fig. 8.4). Third-party payers have formularies, which are set lists of medications they will pay for. The patient will only be responsible for a copay, which is not nearly what the drug would cost out of pocket. Often, a provider will write a prescription for something outside the list, and the patient must pay out of pocket or may need to have the prescription changed to something similar that will be covered on their plan. The pharmacy can request a change on the patient's behalf. In some cases, prior authorization may be required. This process happens when the pharmacy informs the provider and requests documentation based on what the insurance company requires. If the drug is approved, the patient will be able to get the prescription filled for that specific medication. One of the biggest problems with all these scenarios is that the process takes time. The patient may have to wait a week after seeing the provider for the medication to be changed or receive prior approval, and this is often an excuse for nonadherence. They will have to make calls to find out progress and return to the pharmacy for pickup. From the patient's view, this is all additional time and trouble involved in following the treatment plan.

 Tech Note

Nearly half of the approximately 4 billion prescriptions dispensed in the United States each year are not taken as prescribed, according to the *New England Journal of Medicine* (Jimmy & Jose, 2011).

COMPLICATED DOSING OR ADMINISTRATION

For most adult patients, taking the oral-dose form of a medication is the easiest way to adhere to medication administration. Storage is easy and convenient. When the form of medication is an inhaler, injection, or topical application, however, things are more complicated. It's inconvenient to apply something to the skin at work or to find a place to administer an inhaler dose. This causes patients to skip doses or change times to what is most convenient, which affects the processes of how the drug reacts in the body, such as absorption and metabolism. For example, the dose calls for a cream to be applied TID, or three times a day, and the patient works from 8 to 5 daily. The patient chooses to apply the cream once before work and then twice after work in the evening. Instead of a dose every 8 hours, the patient is applying the medication at 7 a.m. and then two doses back to back (3 hours apart) at 6 p.m. and 9 p.m., which may not be optimal. As another example, if a medication requires refrigeration and a refrigerator is not available at the patient's workplace, the medication cannot be stored properly, which may affect its potency.

When the medication requires an injection (e.g., hormones such as testosterone), adherence can be extremely hard for some patients (Fig. 8.5). Not only do they have to overcome the fear of an injection, but they usually must find someone to administer the dose. It may require taking time from work to go to the provider's office weekly or monthly and paying an additional copay. If patients have diabetes and require insulin injections, they must learn to inject themselves daily and adhere to a dosing schedule while trying to maintain a normal routine. Management of diabetes also includes testing their blood glucose and maintaining the additional required supplies needed for testing and injections.

LACK OF RESOURCES

Many patients have limited resources, and often the provider is unaware of the patient's situation. A provider may prescribe a medication and never know if the patient can afford to get it filled. The patient leaves the office with instructions and a medication prescription, and unless there is a problem with the medication or some type of intervention from the pharmacy or

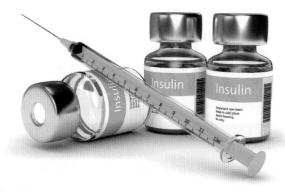

Fig. 8.5 Insulin vials and syringe. (Copyright @ iStock/ayo888.)

another provider, the primary care provider assumes that the instructions are being followed and that the prescription was filled. The patient may be embarrassed to tell the provider that he or she can't afford the medication or can't get the medication for other reasons, such as a lack of transportation.

PERSONAL BELIEFS, RELIGION, OR PERCEPTION

Cultural differences and belief systems are important factors in medication adherence. Many patients perceive diseases, such as those related to mind (e.g., schizophrenia, depression) or behavioral conditions, as embarrassing and often live in turmoil because the diseases are so debilitating. Many of these patients are low functioning and are unable to participate in normal day-to-day activities, such as employment. Gender plays a part as well—most women are more compliant with medication adherence compared with men. Age, marital status, and religious preferences also play a part. Patients with high levels of religious faith sometimes rely on prayer and see taking medications or even vaccines as a sign of weakness or a lack of faith in God. There are also some religions that have specific practices that affect treatment, such as observances of holy days when surgical procedures cannot be done. The Amish believe the heart is "the soul of the body" and do not allow transplants. Some branches of Hinduism restrict the use of any drug or medical dressing that originates from parts of a pig. There are many nuances in this area, and it is important to be informed and respectful of patients' diverse beliefs.

Some may perceive mental illness as negative or as something that can just "be fixed." The stigma associated with mental illness can delay diagnosis or treatment, even though many employers offer counseling that is covered by insurance or free in many cases.

STRATEGIES TO IMPROVE MEDICATION ADHERENCE

Now that we have discussed several barriers to medication adherence, let's discuss some ways advanced technicians can assist in improving adherence or overcoming these barriers. Technicians are often the first contact for a patient at the pharmacy counter. Being the eyes and ears and observing behaviors are key to identifying some early problems. Communicating directly with patients as they drop off new prescriptions or ask for refills and listening to their concerns can be instrumental in identifying times to involve the pharmacist.

INCLUDE PATIENTS IN DECISIONS REGARDING THEIR MEDICATIONS

Approaching medication adherence as a collaborative process opens the door to patients being more involved in their own care and feeling ownership of their conditions. They see other care providers sharing information and including them in decisions rather than just being told what to do. An advanced technician with knowledge of the barriers and the importance of adhering to medication regimens adds another layer of support to the patient and the caregiver team.

Ways to include and support patients in the prescribing process include the following:

- Ensure the patient understands the instructions. Use open-ended questions, such as, "Can you tell me how you have been taking this?" rather than "Have you been taking this once a day?"
- Ensure any additional requests or concerns are shared with the pharmacist, including the offer of counseling. Observe patients' body language when explaining their medications; hesitation, for example, may prompt a counseling offer in some cases.
- Ask patients if they were given any additional instructions by the provider regarding medications, tests, or treatment that they need clarification on.
- If the medication dose form is complicated, such as an inhaler or injection, offer additional information or suggestions. Patients may need to find a provider to administer the injection or may need additional supplies for a caregiver to administer the injections at home, such as syringes or alcohol swabs. In many of today's community pharmacies, there are clinics where injections can be administered on-site. Patients are not always aware of these services and will look to the advanced technician, as their first contact, to provide this information.

COMMUNICATION IMPROVEMENT METHODS

Being thorough and answering any and all questions about medications are key to helping with medication adherence. Taking the time to listen and being clear about any necessary information or adverse effects will remove the unknown from the scenario and provide a basis for compliance. Surprises when taking a new medication are not going to help with adherence. Documentation of any concerns, past issues, or even successes by the advanced technician allows the pharmacist and other providers to monitor progress accurately. Identifying barriers, such as language, for the pharmacist allows the pharmacist to intervene and relieve the patient's worry or clarify information for the patient if needed. For example, if the past refills have not been picked up regularly (on time), this should be noted for the pharmacist because there may be a pattern of missed or skipped doses.

INCORPORATION OF COMMON MEDICATION ADMINISTRATION AIDS

As the front person in a community pharmacy, the advanced technician can offer many aids to the patient to improve adherence (Fig. 8.6). Some of these include:

- Medication calendars
- Medication pamphlets or information sheets
- Medication containers or "pillboxes"
- Special containers such as non-child-proof lids or time-of-dose markings
- Synchronizing medications by use of special packaging such as "unit of use" strips or cards

Many pharmacies offer special packaging with pouches that hold all the medication due at a dose time, such as breakfast, lunch, and dinner (Fig. 8.7). Rather than removing their medication from individual bottles or a pillbox that must be refilled weekly or monthly at home, the pharmacy prepares a month's

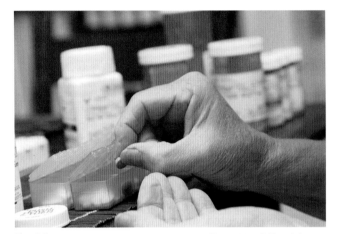

Fig. 8.6 Example of filling weekly pillboxes. (Copyright @ iStock/jorgeantonio.)

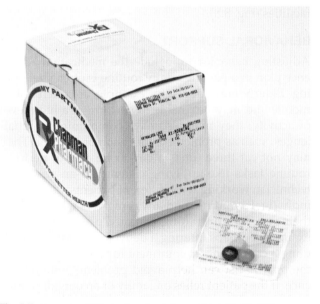

Fig. 8.7 Example of 30-day box for delivery of a patient's strip-packaged medications. (From Davis, K., & Guerra, A. [2019]. *Mosby's pharmacy technician* [5th ed.]. St. Louis, MO: Elsevier.)

💬 **Tech Note**

When assisting with a patient, remember to address the "how, why, what, when, and how long." Knowledge is power, and the more patients understand these elements, the more they will understand the importance of taking care of themselves by adhering to the medication regimen.

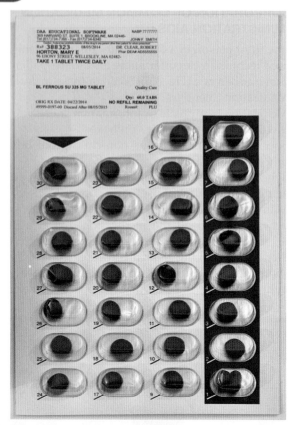

Fig. 8.8 Completed blister pack for 30-day dosing. (From Davis, K., & Guerra, A. [2019]. *Mosby's pharmacy technician* [5th ed.]. St. Louis, MO: Elsevier.)

supply, and the patient just tears each pouch open. Errors are prevented, and adherence is enhanced; additionally, this packaging is easy to transport, and everything is ready from pickup.

If the patient prefers, there are also 30-day cards that can be filled. These are often used in long-term care facilities (Fig. 8.8).

BEHAVIORAL SUPPORT

Adjusting behavior to include the medication adherence plan in a patient's daily routine is often challenging. Elderly individuals, for example, are often not as mobile and may be unable to perform at a high level of activity; they may also have communication challenges, such as problems with vision or hearing. They may not eat three times a day or be able to perform routine tasks like applying creams. As an advanced technician working with different patients, identifying individuals' routines and any caregivers who aid with their care helps in crafting a tailored plan for them. For example, perhaps offering a delivery service or scheduling a counseling appointment for the caregiver with the pharmacist can help avoid problems with adherence. If the patient relies on family or an outside source for help with medication, this should be noted in the patient's record, and that person should be included in the treatment plan for the patient while ensuring that

Health Insurance Portability and Accountability Act (HIPAA) rules are followed.

Going the extra mile, such as providing texts or emails for reminders for refills, special packaging, or instructions in the patient's native language, can assist special populations with medication adherence.

REGULAR FOLLOW-UP/SUPPORTIVE EFFORTS

As important as the initial diagnosis and adherence to the medication program are, monitoring and documentation are also critical. An advanced technician who works closely with the patient, participates in routine refills, and has one-on-one conversations with the patient has many opportunities to assist with supportive efforts. Scheduling refills through reminders, assisting the pharmacist with counseling efforts or appointments, and acting as a liaison and fact-finder for the patient create a team effort and can significantly affect the success of the patient in achieving better health. Indirect supportive efforts, such as pill counts, review of calendars or tests results, and monitoring of timeliness of refills, can be beneficial as well. These are all indicators of medication adherence and can be reported to the pharmacist, who can then provide counseling or other collaborative efforts on the patient's behalf.

CONTINUOUS ASSESSMENT

Today's record-keeping technology is a great tool in a medication adherence program. The determination of rates of refill prescriptions by reviewing the pharmacy's computerized records can offer compliance information. The use of electronic health records (EHRs) can also provide patient treatment information in conjunction with a prescribed medication regimen. These records can be accessed in real time and can be shared with anyone who is participating in the patient's care. EHRs provide an accurate and current picture of the patient and reduce errors such as duplication of therapy. Automatic refill programs, often referred to as *synchronization programs*, encourage the patient to pick up medications at the same time each month. Such programs ensure a routine monthly refill without interruption, along with fewer trips to the pharmacy. At the time of the prescription pickup, programs such as anticoagulation, statin, or thyroid monitoring can also occur. An advanced technician can also schedule appointments, send refill reminders, and document tests or results.

METHODS USED IN ONGOING ASSESSMENT AND MEASUREMENT OF SUCCESS

In today's pharmacy, many advanced technician roles include involvement in **medication reconciliation** programs. The goal of medication reconciliation is to maintain an accurate record of medication for a patient in order to provide for safe and effective use. The Joint Commission has developed five steps in the process

as part of the National Patient Safety Goals https://
www.jointcommission.org/standards/national-
patient-safety-goals/, as follows:

- Develop a list of current prescription medications, including over-the-counter medicines, herbal medicines, and supplements.
- Develop a list of prescribed medications.
- Compare the two lists, looking for duplication of therapy, dosing errors, drug interactions, medication adherence issues, and omission of drugs.
- Make clinical decisions based on this comparison.
- Share the information with any providers and other members of the healthcare team associated with the patient.

THE ADVANCED TECHNICIAN'S ROLE IN MEDICATION RECONCILIATION AND ERROR PREVENTION

Advanced technicians have three roles in medication reconciliation and error prevention:

- Obtaining preadmission medication and health history for the patient
- Working closely with other pharmacies and providers to obtain relevant patient information
- Documenting and maintaining an ongoing and complete medication list

Because the pharmacy technician has direct and routine contact with the patient at the time of new prescription fills or refills, there is a good opportunity to review and update the patient's medication record. This should include allergies or any problems, such as late refills or medications that may have been returned as a result of nonpickup. Many patients do not realize that vitamins or supplements can interfere with the effectiveness of their prescribed medications, and technicians can routinely explain and record possible interactions. Because advanced technicians have a better understanding and working knowledge of medications, such as the usual dose, route, and brand and generic names, they can assist in preventing errors. Obtaining a baseline of information and maintaining it routinely provide current and accurate records for the pharmacist to use when counseling the patient or discussing the plan with other providers.

Past treatments, surgeries, or tests performed are also important to report. The more information that can be obtained, the better the picture the pharmacist will have when reviewing the medication adherence plan. For example, was the patient diagnosed with a chronic illness, and if so, which ones? Were there past hospitalizations related to this illness? Are there current laboratory test results related to this condition?

Once the information is obtained from the patient, the next step may require the technician to reach out to outside providers to verify the information. Another source of information is the EHR. Comparing the different forms of information takes time and organization on the part of the technician but allows

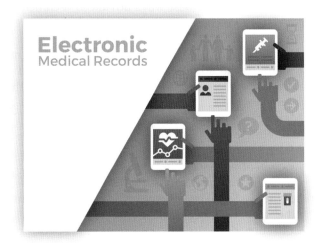

Fig. 8.9 Example electronic health record (EHR). (Copyright @ iStock/filo.)

pharmacists to use their time more efficiently when counseling the patient. Having a complete and accurate history and medication list allows pharmacists to spend the time with the patient on answering questions, explaining and providing interventions, promoting adherence, and making clinical decisions rather than recording and verifying information.

The last step should include a comparison of medications obtained from the admission information, outside sources, and the patient interview to ensure the most accurate medication list is provided to the pharmacist, which will be added to the patient's EHR (Fig. 8.9). The technician and the pharmacist can discuss any discrepancies found or problems that may need to be addressed concerning medication adherence before the pharmacist finalizes the record. For example, perhaps the patient is seeing two physicians, and one has been prescribing Zocor for over a year, whereas the specialist has just started simvastatin. The patient may not realize that one is the generic version of the other and that this is a duplication of medications—they are both statins used for high cholesterol. The technician could bring this to the attention of the pharmacist so that the pharmacist can address the issue with the providers and/or the patient.

USE OF ADVANCED TECHNICIANS IN MEDICATION ADHERENCE PROGRAMS

Advanced technicians who are skilled in direct patient interaction, have good organizational and communication skills, and can pay attention to details can significantly affect a patient's medication adherence. They can identify strategies, help solve problems, and motivate patients with the tools and resources of today's modern and technology-advanced pharmacy.

Along with these responsibilities, technicians can use their existing relationships with patients to motivate and assist patients in taking their medications properly. One of the best ways advanced technicians can assist is to recognize when a patient needs a referral to the pharmacist.

They can also play a primary role by performing many of the administrative duties involved in a medication adherence program, which include the following:

- Making initial appointments for counseling
- Gathering medication histories
- Making reminder calls for refills
- Documenting assessments for patients
- Marketing and promoting the program
- Serving as a liaison between the pharmacy and other team members (providers)
- Collecting demographic information needed for a pharmacist counseling session
- Tracking improvements and maintaining outcomes through electronic methods
- Conducting follow-up surveys on patient satisfaction
- Filling synchronized medications
- Managing follow-up calls and requests from patients

Medication nonadherence is a widespread issue. Encouraging adherence to a plan involves a multidisciplinary approach, with pharmacy, medical providers, and clinical and supportive personnel working with the patient in support of the patient's goals (Fig. 8.10). Each branch of practice should work toward enhancing a patient's overall health and use the expertise and knowledge of their areas of practice. Pharmacy technicians will continue to be used in more clinical roles and are thus positioned to greatly influence the services that are provided to patients. This will advance healthcare and improve patient safety.

Case Study

You are working with a patient to update her medication reconciliation plan. The patient states that she recently moved from out of town and lost all her medications in the move. She has diabetes and sees three providers regularly.

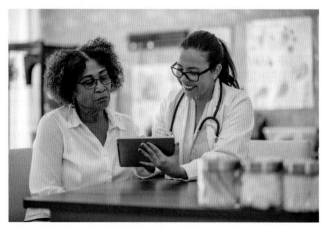

Fig. 8.10 A technician interviewing a patient and gathering medication history electronically. (Copyright @ iStock/FatCamera.)

What would be the best approach to get the most accurate information needed to complete the patient's plan?

Ask for the providers' contact information.

Ask for any third-party information (the patient may have a current list of her medications or contact information for the pharmacy that last filled the prescriptions).

Ask if there is anyone assisting the patient with her medication who might have more information.

Ask where she previously got her prescriptions filled.

Record when she last took her medications, especially those related to diabetes.

Contact any outside sources if provided.

Discuss next steps with the pharmacist once as much information as can be obtained is recorded.

REVIEW QUESTIONS

1. Which of the following terms describes the condition of a patient with diabetes who requires ongoing medication and treatment?
   a. Acute condition
   b. Continuous condition
   c. Chronic condition
   d. None of the above

2. Which of the following terms describes the condition of a patient who suddenly gets strep throat and requires medication?
   a. Acute condition
   b. Continuous condition
   c. Chronic condition
   d. None of the above

3. Patients are said to be adherent to therapy if they take their prescribed medication at least _____ of the time.
   a. 70%
   b. 65%
   c. 75%
   d. 80%

4. Which of the following diseases is reported to not be controlled sufficiently in adults between the ages of 35 and 64?
   a. Hypertension
   b. COPD
   c. Diabetes
   d. Mental health disease

5. Which of the following diseases is referred to as the "silent killer"?
   a. Hypertension
   b. COPD
   c. Diabetes
   d. Mental health disorder

6. Which of the following medication adherence terms best describes a patient starting a medication but stopping it before a healthcare professional advises it?
   a. Nonpersistence
   b. Nonfulfillment
   c. Nonconformance
   d. Nonadherence

7. Which medication adherence term describes a patient who takes medication at the wrong times or skips doses?
   a. Nonpersistence
   b. Nonfulfillment
   c. Nonconformance
   d. Nonadherence
8. Which organization has developed National Patient Safety Goals that include medication reconciliation requirements?
   a. The Joint Commission
   b. CMS
   c. HHS
   d. None of the above
9. All of the following are common duties performed by technicians in a medication adherence program EXCEPT:
   a. Creating medication lists
   b. Tracking outcomes
   c. Counseling patients
   d. Filling synchronized medications
10. When preparing an admission history for a patient in the medication reconciliation process, which of the following should be noted for the pharmacist if found?
    a. Drug interactions
    b. Refills not picked up
    c. Dosing errors
    d. All of the above

CRITICAL THINKING QUESTIONS

1. You are interviewing a patient to gather a medication history, and you find that the patient is complaining about having to come several times each month to get the medications. What would you suggest, and how would you explain the service's benefits?
2. Discuss ways that medication adherence benefits the public.

REFERENCES

American Heart Association. (2020). The Facts about High Blood Pressure Retrieved November 1, 2019 from https://www.heart.org/en/health-topics/high-blood-pressure/the-facts-about-high-blood-pressure.

Benjamin, R. M. (2012). Medication adherence: helping patients take their medicines as directed. Public health reports (Washington, D.C. : 1974), *127*(1), 2–3. https://doi.org/10.1177/003335491212700102.

Jimmy, B., & Jose, J. (2011). Patient medication adherence: measures in daily practice. *Oman medical journal, 26*(3), 155–159. https://doi.org/10.5001/omj.2011.38.

Kadia, N. K., & Schroeder, M. N. (2015). Community Pharmacy–Based Adherence Programs and the Role of Pharmacy Technicians: A Review. *Journal of Pharmacy Technology, 31*(2), 51–57. https://doi.org/10.1177/8755122515572809.

9 | Sterile Products and Hazardous Drugs

Learning Objectives

1. Discuss the history of chapters 797 and 800 of the *United States Pharmacopeia* and their impact on today's pharmacy practices.
2. Discuss required training, environmental control, and other responsibilities for advanced technicians working with nonhazardous and hazardous sterile products.
3. Identify common responsibilities for advanced technicians in roles associated with sterile compounding.

Key Terms

Aseptic technique Procedure used to prevent contamination of compounded sterile preparations (CSPs).

Beyond-use date (BUD) Date assigned at time of compounding, after which the product should no longer be used and be discarded.

Compounded sterile preparation (CSP) Medication prepared using the sterile compounding processes.

Compounding record (CR) Document (recipe) used to record processes and drugs used to prepare a specific patient's compounded sterile preparation (CSP).

Garbing Donning or putting on personal protective equipment (PPE) in a required series of steps.

Gloved fingertip and thumb sampling Personnel test used to determine whether any microorganisms are present on hands.

ISO Class 5 area Designated environment for primary engineering control (PEC) used in compounding sterile medications.

ISO Class 7 area Designated area for primary engineering control (PEC) to be kept; also known as a *clean room* or *anteroom*.

ISO Class 8 area Designated area for handwashing and garbing to take place in; also known as a *buffer room*.

Master formula record (MFR) Document (recipe) of the processes and medications used in preparing a compounded sterile preparation (CSP).

Media fill testing A test of a prepared compounded sterile preparation (CSP) used to determine the aseptic technique of compounding personnel with the use of a media growth product.

Standard operating procedure (SOP) Set of procedures used to ensure sterility of all compounded sterile preparations (CSPs).

Sterile Free of living organisms.

Surface sampling Test performed to determine whether microorganisms are present on surfaces in sterile environment areas.

INTRODUCTION

Sterile compounding is traditionally being performed in today's pharmacy by technicians who have received additional training in **aseptic technique** (Fig. 9.1). Several organizations have established regulations or guidelines for all aspects of the process, and the US Pharmacopeia (USP) recently updated its guidelines. These guidelines are acknowledged by state boards of pharmacy, the American Society of Health-System Pharmacists (ASHP), The Joint Commission, and other related organizations as the standards of practice. For pharmacy technicians who wish to seek a specialty or advanced role in sterile compounding, it is important to know the guidelines and have a heightened sense of the responsibility involved in preparing these types of medications.

The **compounded sterile preparations (CSPs)** affected by the updated USP regulations include several types of sterile compounds broken into two categories: Category 1, which includes CSPs that have an assigned **beyond-use date (BUD)** of less than 12 hours at room temperature or 24 hours or less if refrigerated, and Category 2, those CSPs assigned a BUD of more than 12 hours at room temperature and 24 hours or greater if refrigerated. The factors used to determine the category include the following:
- Conditions they are made in
- Probability of bacterial growth
- Time period they will be used for

The USP guidelines are designed to prevent contamination through practices and environmental quality and to ensure the sterility of the final CSPs made. These CSPs may be for human or animal use.

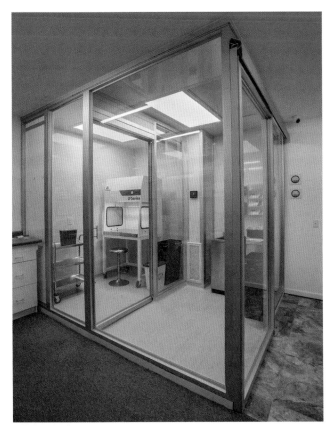

Fig. 9.1 Intravenous (IV) room. (From Davis, K. [2020]. *Mosby's sterile compounding for pharmacy technicians* [2nd ed.]. St. Louis, MO: Elsevier.)

The most common form is injectable, but other forms include the following:
- Aqueous (water-based CSPs, e.g., bronchial inhalations)
- Live organ baths and soaks
- Ophthalmic medications
- Internal body cavity irrigations

OVERVIEW OF CHAPTER 797 PHARMACEUTICAL COMPOUNDING—STERILE PREPARATIONS

- The USP recently updated chapter 797 of the *United States Pharmacopeia* to reflect updated practices and guidelines. These guidelines were written by experts in the field and made available to practitioners and the public for review. The most recent version was made available in June 2019 and is pending official release. The purpose of chapter 797 is to identify best-practice guidelines for sterile compounding, and the guidelines are enforced by many organizations. Chapter 797 provides guidelines that ensure positive outcomes for patient safety by providing policies and procedures that will accomplish this. Some of the sections include the following:
- Personnel training, including handwashing and **garbing**

- Environmental controls
- Documentation, labeling, storage, and disposal
- Quality control and quality assurance plans

CHAPTER 797 GUIDELINES FOR PERSONNEL TRAINING

Guidelines for handwashing and garbing are provided in chapter 797, and personnel must be trained and evaluated at least yearly to assess performance (Fig. 9.2).

Handwashing and garbing instructions include washing the hands following the recommendations of the Centers for Disease Control and Prevention (CDC), along with a series of steps for garbing, as follows: Put on shoe covers, head cover, and facial cover, followed by a face mask. Perform handwashing. Put on nonshedding gown and sterile gloves (Fig. 9.3).

As an advanced technician working with other technicians in compounding facilities, you may serve to evaluate adherence to these processes by observation. This should be accomplished by following a **standard operating procedure (SOP)** that the facility has created. The SOP may have step-by-step instructions, and evaluations will need to be maintained in the employee's records. Personnel who compound must be observed yearly for their actual technique and finished products and reevaluated if not successful.

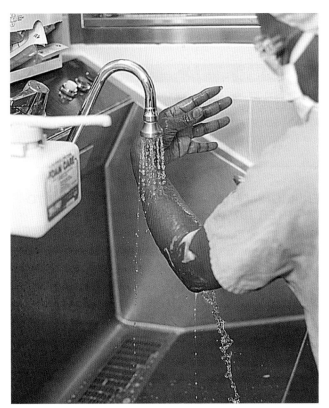

Fig. 9.2 Handwashing. (From Davis, K., & Guerra, A. [2019]. *Mosby's pharmacy technician* [5th ed.]. St. Louis, MO: Elsevier.)

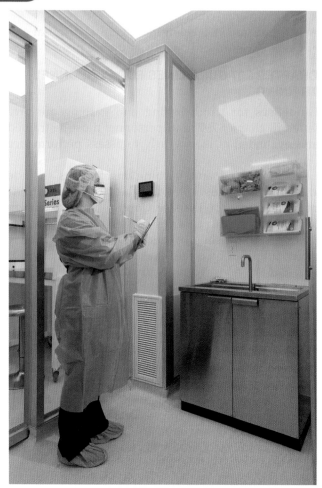

Fig. 9.3 Technician garbed and ready to perform sterile compounding. (From Davis, K. [2020]. *Mosby's sterile compounding for pharmacy technicians* [2nd ed.]. St. Louis, MO: Elsevier.)

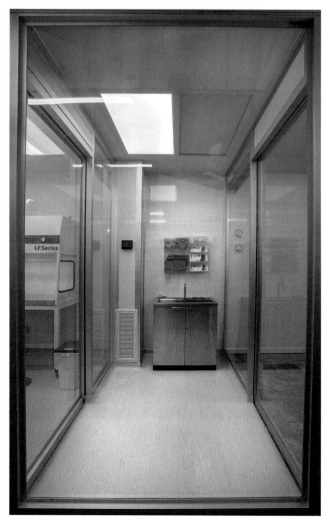

Fig. 9.4 Buffer room with sink. (From Davis, K. [2020]. *Mosby's sterile compounding for pharmacy technicians* [2nd ed.]. St. Louis, MO: Elsevier.)

 Tech Note

According to the CDC, handwashing reduces diarrheal illness in people with weakened immune systems by 58% (CDC, 2019). Most patients requiring sterile medications have compromised immune systems as a result of trauma, illness, or other conditions (CDC, 2019).

ENVIRONMENTAL CONTROLS ACCORDING TO CHAPTER 797

The chapter 797 guidelines provide a clear picture of the environment required for sterile compounding. This includes supplies, equipment, air quality, temperature, and storage (Fig. 9.4). The spaces include two distinct areas where certain tasks must take place.

One is the anteroom, or **International Organization for Standards (ISO) Class 8 area**; this is where the sink is placed and where handwashing and garbing take place. This area is designed to be used prior to entering the next cleanest area, which is the buffer room or **ISO Class 7 area**. Entering this space requires personnel to be appropriately garbed. Once inside the Class 7 area, there is a dedicated space or primary engineering control (PEC)

where the actual CSPs are prepared using aseptic technique. This is the **ISO Class 5 area** in the form of a "hood." This can be a laminar airflow workspace (LAFW), a laminar airflow system (LAFS), or a restricted-access barrier system (RABS) (Figs. 9.5 and 9.6).

These areas require constant monitoring of temperature and humidity to avoid the growth of microorganisms in the environment. The temperature should be 68°F, and the humidity should be maintained at 60%. Both types of PECs also use a high-efficiency particulate air (HEPA) filter to ensure air quality. Maintenance of a clean environment is an important task that technicians must perform. This includes daily cleaning of floors, counters, and work surfaces. Walls and ceilings are cleaned monthly, and the PECs are cleaned more frequently based on their use. These processes must be recorded on a log and kept as part of the facility's SOP documentation. In addition, **surface sampling** must occur periodically to ensure the cleaning procedures have been done correctly. This entails taking a sample of the surface quarterly using a device such as a sterile cotton

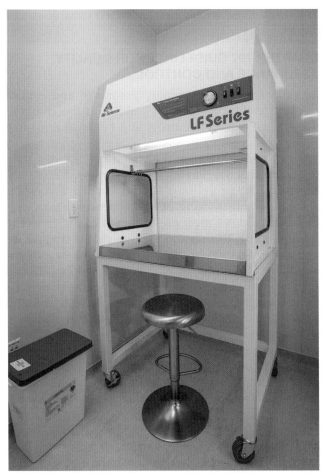

Fig. 9.5 Laminar airflow workspace (LAFW; primary engineering control [PEC]) in a pharmacy. (From Davis, K. [2020]. *Mosby's sterile compounding for pharmacy technicians* [2nd ed.]. St. Louis, MO: Elsevier.)

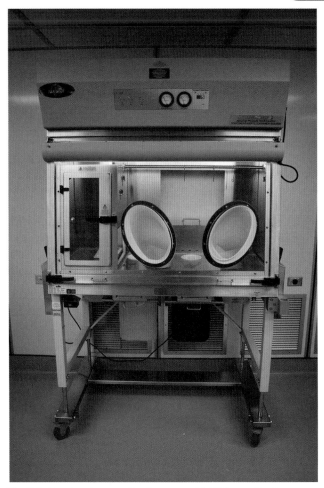

Fig. 9.6 Restricted-access barrier system (RABS), specifically, a compounding aseptic isolator (CACI). (Courtesy CriticalPoint, LLC, Totowa, New Jersey.)

swab and placing it on an agar plate. This plate is then incubated to allow any bacteria to grow if present.

The facility must ensure the PECs and the environment have a current certificate of analysis (COA) provided by an authorized outside company. This is done every 6 months and validates the air quality and microbial sterility of the area.

The compounding person must also adhere to proper hand placement to avoid blocking the horizontal airflow across critical sites, such as vial tops or needle hubs. Training for proper technique includes yearly observation of handwashing, garbing, and aseptic technique and a **gloved fingertip and thumb sampling** every 6 months. This is performed by placing the fingers and thumbs on an agar plate and incubating the plate to allow bacteria to grow if present. The presence of bacterial growth would indicate improper handwashing and garbing procedures, and the operator would need remediation. The sterility of finished CSPs is validated through a process called **media fill testing**. Testing of a final compound every 6 months with the use of growth media demonstrates that the product is free of pyrogens and bacteria. This can only be accomplished if the compounder uses proper aseptic technique.

DOCUMENTATION, STORAGE, AND DISPOSAL PER CHAPTER 797 GUIDELINES

Many of the advanced technician roles in today's pharmacy include maintaining and tracking formulas using advanced technology. The use of specific forms includes a **master formula record (MFR)**. The MFR is used to record the procedures and items required to compound a specific CSP. It can be used like a "recipe" and must be included as part of the pharmacy's records. In addition, each compound prepared for a patient must be recorded on a **compounding record (CR)**. This ensures that there is a way to track the product and all its components or "ingredients" if there are recalls, adverse effects, or other reasons to trace the compound to the patient or facility.

As part of the process of documenting a CSP, there must be an assignment of a BUD. This is different from the expiration date, which is provided by the manufacturer if the product is maintained in its original packaging. The BUD is generally shorter and takes into account the preparation or mixing of ingredients. It can also include the storage form that the final product will use. For example, a CSP in the form of an intravenous (IV) bag is made of normal saline with cefazolin added. The vial of cefazolin is taken from its original container, reconstituted, and added to the bag of fluid. Because of this preparation process, the final prepared bag is assigned a BUD of 4 days if refrigerated. This is based on the manufacturer's recommendations of a missed product found in pharmacy reference materials.

Disposal of unused sterile products requires knowledge of current USP guidelines, along with Occupational Safety and Health Administration (OSHA) guidelines for workplace safety and the Environmental Protection Agency (EPA) regulations for environmental concerns. Expired or waste CSPs must be placed in a blue and white plastic container and properly disposed of by incineration. Sharp objects, such as needles or broken vials or ampules, must be placed in red containers (Fig. 9.7). Some medications also require special disposal, such as live vaccines, which are considered hazardous and require a special purple container.

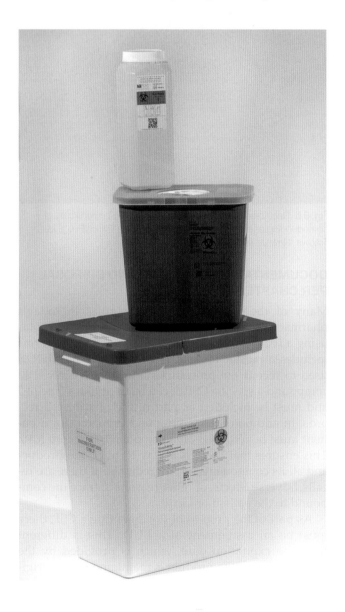

Fig. 9.7 Various waste containers. (From Davis, K. [2020]. *Mosby's sterile compounding for pharmacy technicians* [2nd ed.]. St. Louis, MO: Elsevier.)

CHAPTER 797 GUIDELINES FOR QUALITY ASSURANCE AND CONTROL

In today's pharmacy, quality assurance and control are key to the organization's ability to be competitive and efficient while providing the most error-free sterile products to patients. A quality assurance (QA) program should include SOPs and policies designed to ensure that the facility's predetermined goals are achieved. QA procedures should include a constant evaluation and tracking of best practices, along with those that did not meet preset requirements. In sterile compounding, this should include results from training and evaluation of personnel, maintenance of environmental controls, availability of medications and supplies, and completion of proper documentation. As an advanced technician, the review of a QA plan and subsequent collaboration with other team members and supervisory personnel can lead to changes that result in improved patient safety and overall efficiency.

Quality control (QC) involves using the information gathered from an active QA program to assess quality and make changes to processes. This could include the following:

- Setting up additional training for personnel based on observations or other validation testing
- Reassigning personnel responsibilities to consider proper assignment or alignment of duties
- Rearranging workflow processes, such as making changes to spaces, order of tasks, or time allotted to tasks (see Chapter 5)
- Reviewing current uses of technology or automation and considering changes if appropriate
- Determining whether streamlining business or billing processes could improve services provided
- Determining how drug shortages affect patient care and creating proactive ways to eliminate barriers

Case Study

As the coordinator for a large compounding facility, you are asked to help the facility prepare for a state board of pharmacy inspection that is coming up soon. What type of documentation would you gather? Are there any additional tasks that you would want to do before the visit?

The inspector will be looking at several items, including the following:

- Current and new-hire initial and recertification training documents
- Examples of completed media fill test results
- Documentation of observation of personnel performing handwashing, garbing, and aseptic technique
- Cleaning logs

- Surface sample test results
- Gloved fingertip/thumb test results
- Routine checks for temperature and humidity of environment (logs)
- Written SOPs
- Current certificates of analysis for the PECs and environment
- Samples of completed CR and MFR records to match dispensed CSPs

Additional tasks may include a review to ensure all documents are available for inspection and are up to date.

CHAPTER 800 HAZARDOUS PHARMACEUTICALS GUIDELINES

The latest revision of chapter 800 of the *United States Pharmacopeia* became effective December 1, 2019. This chapter was previously incorporated in chapter 797, and the general requirements for nonhazardous CSPs should be followed, with a few differences. The drugs considered to be hazardous drugs (HDs) are determined by the National Institute for Occupational Safety and Health (NIOSH). The most common forms seen in hazardous sterile compounding are chemotherapy drugs used to treat cancer and radiopharmaceuticals. When performing handwashing and garbing for procedures involving HDs, the donning of gloves is different. Special, thicker gloves and double gloving are required for HDs. The environmental controls are not the same. The containment primary engineering control (C-PEC) for preparing sterile HDs is usually a biological safety cabinet (BSC) (Fig. 9.8).

This "hood" has vertical airflow rather than horizontal, so operators are not exposed to air coming straight across the work surface toward them. In addition, CSP chemotherapy waste should be placed in a yellow plastic container inside the BSC. Other medications listed as hazardous are disposed of in a black plastic container. The use of a chemo or preparation mat on the work surface of the C-PEC is required to catch and absorb any spills while preparing the CSP. Disposal of all contaminated waste (anything used while preparing the CSP inside the C-PEC), including garbing materials, should be disposed of in a marked hazardous waste container.

The withdrawal of fluid from a vial requires the use of a closed-system transfer device (CSTD). This is a vented spike device that eliminates the use of a needle and lessens the chance of spray.

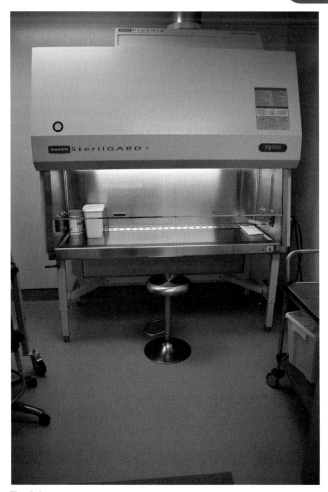

Fig. 9.8 Biological safety cabinet (BSC). (Courtesy CriticalPoint, LLC, Totowa, New Jersey.)

RESPONSIBILITIES OF ADVANCED TECHNICIANS IN STERILE COMPOUNDING ROLES

Many of today's compounding pharmacy responsibilities are being performed by technicians, and with the number of patients needing sterile compounds, the need for proper technique and training cannot be ignored. In many cases, facilities are requiring advanced technicians to have national certification (certified pharmacy technician [CPhT]) and additional specialty training, such as the certified compounded sterile preparation technician (CSPT) certification offered by the Pharmacy Technician Certification Board (PTCB), in order to work in this area. There are also many opportunities to serve in coordinator roles. The operation of the department and daily workflow affect patients directly, in addition to the other healthcare providers who treat the patient simultaneously. Adherence to guidelines and regulations must be managed, including all elements being in compliance with chapters 797 and 800 of the *United States Pharmacopeia* and with the regulations of state boards of pharmacy. This requires constant attention and periodic evaluations, including the following:

- Routine sampling of environment (daily)
- Cleaning routine (daily, monthly)

Tech Note

Each year, about 200 million adults needing medical intervention in the United States have an IV line inserted into their arm to deliver vital fluids, nutrients, and medicines (ICT, 2017).

- New-employee training
- Recertification of employees through written tests, observation, and final testing or validation
- Completion of documentation and written procedures as needed (MFR, CR, and new SOPs)

The advanced technician with additional training in sterile compounding can play a key role in the services provided to patients. Pharmacists who can rely on advanced technicians with an understanding of industry guidelines and regulations regarding sterile compounding are able to use their time for direct clinical support of the patient. Working as a team toward patient-centered care must involve everyone associated with the patient. Capitalizing on the strengths of technicians with specialty training in sterile compounding provides another level of expertise and quality.

REVIEW QUESTIONS

1. Which of the following chapters is associated with hazardous sterile compounding?
   a. ASHP 797
   b. ASHP 800
   c. *United States Pharmacopeia* 800
   d. *United States Pharmacopeia* 797
2. Which of the following chapters is associated with compounding of sterile nonhazardous products?
   a. ASHP 797
   b. ASHP 800
   c. *United States Pharmacopeia* 800
   d. *United States Pharmacopeia* 797
3. The processes used to prepare sterile compounds are referred to as which of the following?
   a. Master technique
   b. Compounding technique
   c. Aseptic technique
   d. None of the above
4. Which area is designated for handwashing and garbing procedures?
   a. ISO Class 5
   b. ISO Class 7
   c. ISO Class 8
   d. PEC
5. Which area is designated for aseptic technique?
   a. ISO Class 5
   b. ISO Class 7

   c. ISO Class 8
   d. PEC
6. Which of the following is an acceptable type of PEC in which HDs can be prepared?
   a. BSC
   b. LAFW
   c. LAFS
   d. RABS
7. Which of the following best describes the form used to record a specific patient's CSP once prepared?
   a. MFR
   b. CR
   c. SOP
   d. None of the above
8. Which of the following would be the best way to determine the sterility of a final CSP?
   a. Media fill testing
   b. Gloved fingertip/thumb testing
   c. Surface sampling
   d. Observation of aseptic technique
9. Which container would be appropriate for the disposal of used gowns, gloves, and spill mats used in preparing a chemotherapy CSP?
   a. Yellow
   b. Red
   c. Purple
   d. Blue and white
10. When preparing an HD CSP, which of the following should be used?
    a. CSTD
    b. Spill mat
    c. Double gloves
    d. All of the above

CRITICAL THINKING QUESTIONS

1. As the coordinator for a large compounding facility, you are asked to observe the personnel in the IV room today. What would be some specific things you would look for when observing their handwashing and garbing procedures?
2. You are teaching a recertification class on HD preparation today. How would you explain the reasons for and benefits of the use of a CSTD?

REFERENCES

Centers for Disease Control and Prevention. Clean Hands Saves Lives. Retrieved December 10, 2019 from https://www.cdc.gov/handwashing/index.html.

Infection Control Today. New research on IV Infection Risks. Retrieved December 11, 2017 from https://www.infectioncontroltoday.com/infusion-vascular-access/new-research-iv-infection-risk.

Controlled Substance Diversion and Tracking

10

Learning Objectives

1. Discuss the most common controlled substances abused and the need for tracking and prevention guidelines.
2. List the various organizations and states involved and the tracking requirements used in pharmacy today, along with future initiatives.
3. Explain the effects of diversion and drug abuse on society and the public.
4. Discuss the advanced technician's role in the prevention of controlled substance diversion and in tracking programs.

Key Terms

Acute pain Pain that usually starts suddenly and lasts less than 3 months.

Chronic pain Pain, usually caused by a condition or disease, that lasts more than 3 months.

Drug addiction Occurs when attempts to cut back or control use of a controlled substance are unsuccessful.

Drug diversion Any means that deviates the course of a prescription drug from the manufacturer to the intended patient.

Drug misuse Any use of drugs in a manner not directed by a physician.

Drug overdose Injury to the body when a drug is taken in excessive amounts; can be fatal or nonfatal.

Illicit drugs Nonmedical use of a variety of drugs that are prohibited by law, such as cocaine or heroin.

Opiates Natural opioids such as heroin, morphine, and codeine.

Opioid Natural, semisynthetic, or synthetic opioids.

Opioid use disorder (OUD) A chronic disorder featuring a pattern of compulsive opioid use leading to increased tolerance, drug-seeking behaviors, and a failure to fulfill obligations at home, work, or school. Previously known as *drug addiction*.

Prescription Drug Monitoring Program (PDMP) State or territorial electronic databases that track controlled substance prescriptions.

INTRODUCTION

The number of deaths resulting from opioid overdoses has risen significantly since the 1990s (Fig. 10.1). Understanding the epidemic and how to prevent the continued rise is a goal of the Centers for Disease Control and Prevention (CDC) and other agencies, as well as individual states. According to the CDC, more than 700,000 people have died from **drug overdoses** since 1999, and approximately 70% of those deaths were related to opioids. Pharmacies and all healthcare providers today must be active in the prevention of opioid-related harm and increasing public awareness. Advanced technicians can play a significant part in the monitoring, reporting, and patient awareness activities implemented across the country.

OPIOIDS AND COMMON TERMINOLOGY USED IN ASSOCIATION WITH OPIOID ADDICTION

Over 100 million prescriptions for opioids used to treat pain were dispensed in 2017, and that number continues to grow. An **opioid** is a chemical that interacts with receptors in the body or brain to reduce the signal of feelings of pain. An **opiate** is a subset of the broader group of opioids, referring specifically to substances derived from the natural source, that is, the poppy plant. Examples of opiates are heroin, morphine, or codeine. Semisynthetic opioids are created in the laboratory from opiates. Examples include hydromorphone, hydrocodone, and oxycodone. Synthetic opioids are entirely artificial, made in the laboratory to mimic the chemical structure of the opiate. Examples of synthetic opioids are tramadol, methadone, and fentanyl.

All types of opioids have legitimate clinical uses, and all types can be abused.

Opioids are generally safe if taken for short periods of time following an event such as surgery to treat **acute pain**. They may be dispensed to treat pain that is the result of an injury or surgery, and the healing process usually is completed within 3 months. For patients experiencing **chronic pain** or pain that lasts for more than 3 months as a result of a condition such as arthritis, inflammation, or some other disease, opioids can also be prescribed (Fig. 10.2).

The most common drugs in this group are as follows:
- Oxycodone
- Hydrocodone
- Codeine
- Morphine
- Fentanyl

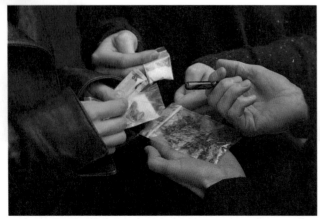

Fig. 10.1 Abuse of drugs is an epidemic. (Copyright © iStock.com/KatarzynanBialasiewicz.)

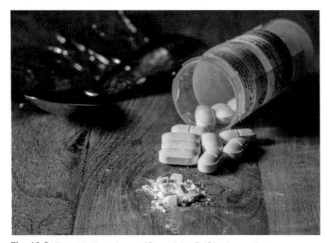

Fig. 10.2 Prescription abuse. (Copyright © iStock.com/BackyardProduction.)

Treating moderate to severe pain is the most common reason for the use of an opioid, but in some cases, pain from cancer, osteoarthritis, or long-term chronic conditions may be treated with opioids. These may include Crohn's disease, chronic obstructive pulmonary disease (COPD), or cystitis fibrosis, for example. With the increase in life expectancy, which has created a larger older adult population, there are more people experiencing these conditions. This has caused a rise in prescription use for this class of drugs and an increase in drug misuse, which is when someone does not follow a provider's directions and overuses the medication by taking it more often than prescribed or taking it in greater amounts than prescribed; it can also occur when someone takes another individual's medication rather than the person it was prescribed for. Opioid use and misuse can result in a tolerance to or dependence on the drug, as well as addiction; the related terms are defined as follows:

Opioid dependence: The body adjusts normal functions with the opioid present, and if the opioid is removed, physical symptoms can occur, such as withdrawal.

Opioid tolerance: When a person is taking opioids and begins to take more and more of the medication to produce the same effects.

opioid use disorder (OUD): The person feels that he or she needs the medication to function normally, and it begins to be too hard to reduce the dose or stop the opioid. The person's daily activities are affected, such as at home and at work.

Physical dependence can result in many symptoms if the medication is stopped or removed, and anyone who takes opioids runs the risk of becoming addicted to them. Individuals may experience withdrawal symptoms when trying to stop or reduce the use of opioids, such as the following:

- Depression
- Increased sensitivity to pain
- Dizziness
- Constipation
- Confusion
- Itching and sweating

The unpleasant effects of the process of stopping opioid use make it extremely hard to convince the person to stop the opioid use. Even once physical detoxification is complete, psychological changes persist, drastically increasing the chances the individual will return to the drug. However, if the individual continues on this path, it can lead to an overdose and death, usually as a result of respiratory failure. Prevention before addiction occurs is the key to managing opioid treatment.

 Tech Note

An **opiate** is a natural form of an opioid, such as heroin, morphine, or codeine.

HEROIN ADDICTION

Heroin is a highly addictive drug made from morphine and extracted from poppy plants. Persons who are addicted to opioids run a high risk of becoming addicted to heroin. Other risk factors include the following:

- Male gender
- Non-Hispanic white ethnicity
- 18- to 25-year-old age range

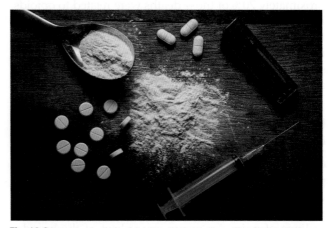

Fig. 10.3 Heroin ready for injection and snorting. (Copyright © iStock.com/wombatzaa.)

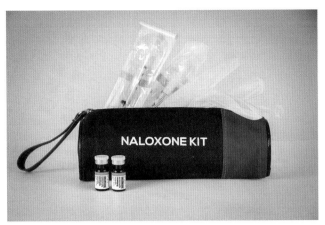

Fig. 10.4 Naloxone kit. (Copyright © iStock.com/NewGig86.)

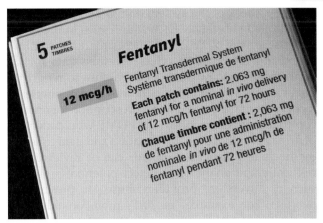

Fig. 10.5 Fentanyl patch label. (Copyright © iStock.com/RobertDupuis.)

- People living in large cities
- People without insurance or medication coverage

Because heroin can be snorted, injected, or smoked, there is also a group of secondary conditions associated with its use (Fig. 10.3). Heroin users may experience long-term viral infections (e.g., human immunodeficiency virus [HIV], hepatitis) and blood- or skin-related diseases.

Medication-assisted treatment (MAT) is generally what is required to treat heroin addiction. This is a combined approach of therapy; counseling; and medication such as methadone, buprenorphine, or naltrexone. Naloxone, delivered via injection, is a life-saving drug that can reverse the effects of an opioid overdose if given in time. Many pharmacies, public entities, and first responders (e.g., police officers and emergency medical services [EMS]) now keep naloxone kits on hand and can administer them per their state laws (Fig. 10.4).

Nonopioid therapy or management of pain can include acupuncture; physical therapy; meditation; exercise; or other medications, such as over-the-counter analgesics. The use of acetaminophen or ibuprofen can provide a way to manage pain without the danger of misuse or overuse of an opioid.

FENTANYL ADDICTION

Fentanyl is a synthetic form of opioid and is many times stronger than morphine. It is generally used for the treatment of advanced cancer or severe pain. It can be dispensed in patches, as lozenges, or by injection. Patches are impregnated with the drug and can have residual drug left on them after disposal (Fig. 10.5). Because of its potency and its relative ease to manufacture, there has been a significant increase in the illegal production of this drug. The euphoric effects are enhanced if it is mixed with cocaine and heroin, and this is appealing to users. Fentanyl is often added to cocaine or heroin on the street to disguise the lower grades of the products being sold as high grade. This is extremely dangerous, as fentanyl overdoses can occur rapidly causing death and the user never knows what they had.

 Tech Note

More than 399,000 people died from overdoses involving any opioid, including prescription and illicit opioids, from 1999 to 2017 (Scholl et al., 2018).

ORGANIZATIONAL STRATEGIES TO COMBAT THE OPIOID CRISIS

The federal government sees the opioid problem as an epidemic and has expanded funding to the US Department of Health and Human Services (HHS 2019). The HHS has a five-point strategy approach that includes the following:

- Better data
- Better pain treatment
- More services related to addiction
- More overdose reversers (naloxone)
- Better research

Other organizations, such as the CDC, have joined the fight by supporting states and communities in the effort. The focus is on identifying outbreaks, collecting data, responding to overdoses, and partnering with public safety officers to battle the growing problem. Widespread awareness and collaboration are encouraged as well.

PRESCRIPTION DRUG MONITORING PROGRAMS

One very significant effort that will be seen in a pharmacy is the state-driven **Prescription Drug Monitoring Program (PDMP)**, which is a statewide electronic database that collects data on prescribed controlled substances. The National Association of State Controlled Substances Authorities (NASCSA) provides specific information for each state at http://www.nascsa.org/rxMonitoring.htm. Currently, 49 states, the District of Columbia, and the US territory of Guam have existing PDMPs.

The benefits of PDMPs continue to grow because information can be shared by providers, and potential abuse or diversion can be prevented. Some states require a check of the system data prior to dispensing a controlled substance. Each state varies in the access and use of the PDMP, but such programs continue to expand. The system offers real-time data for the pharmacist's review, such as the ability to report the patient's prescription history in less than 5 minutes in most cases. If the patient had a prescription for another controlled substance filled, the PDMP would alert the pharmacist at that time. Information and data collected on the state's dispensed opioids can be reviewed periodically and analyzed to detect potential problems, such as diversion, provider abuse, or prescription overuse. For example, in 2017, more opioids were prescribed in Alabama than any other state (over three times as many as those prescribed in the lowest state, Hawaii). What would cause this? Is it related to economics, race, or health status/lifestyle? This is the sort of information that PDMPs can provide for research purposes (Scholl et al., 2018).

EFFECTS ON PUBLIC SAFETY AND COST OF DIVERSION

The use of another person's prescription is one common form of abuse or misuse, but the occurrence of **drug diversion** among healthcare workers is a huge problem as well. The estimated cost of controlled prescription drug diversion and abuse to both public and private medical insurers is approximately $72 billion a year (Lindsay, 2016). The most common drugs stolen are opioids, and this not only affects the healthcare providers' personal health but also that of the patients who do not receive the medication; it also results in unnecessary costs to the public.

Healthcare facilities and organizations spend millions of dollars on systems and preventive measures to develop programs to detect, combat, and deal with confirmed cases. This is costly to the organization and to the public in general. Each case is a loss of product and revenue and affects the overall health of the population. The loss of productivity for workers, the time and monies spent on legal consequences, and increases in drug costs as a result of shrinkage all must be considered. Even society in general feels the sting because the costs related to drug-related crimes, motor vehicle accidents, life insurance premiums, and health insurance premiums all must increase to compensate for the losses. It is estimated that approximately 10% to 15% of pharmacists, nurses, and physicians are potential substance abusers.

OTHER INITIATIVES THAT BENEFIT THE PUBLIC

As an advanced pharmacy technician, there will be opportunities to assist patients in making safer choices regarding their prescriptions. Medicine take-back programs are very popular all over the country, and companies such as Walgreens have medication disposal kiosks or mailbox-type boxes where unwanted medications

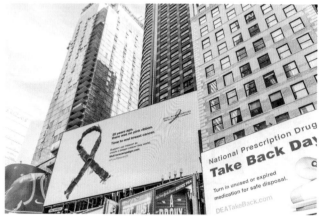

Fig. 10.6 Take Back Drug sign in New York City. (Copyright © iStock. com/krblokhin.)

can be placed for disposal. The US Drug Enforcement Agency (DEA) also has National Prescription Drug Take-Back Days in April and October, and the public is encouraged to dispose of unwanted drugs on these days so that they can be safely disposed of (Fig. 10.6). Leaving these around the house can tempt some to misuse them, especially controlled drugs, and there is also the danger of accidental ingestion by children. The DEA also offers an RX Abuse Online Reporting program that is designed for anonymous reporting of abuse (see https://apps2.deadiversion.usdoj.gov/rxaor/spring/main?execution=e1s1).

Proper disposal of medications because of expiration or nonuse keeps these from being available for abuse and protects the public. It is much safer if these medications are disposed of rather than left around the home. Technicians have frequent opportunities for one-on-one conversations with patients. Review the scenarios in the following case studies and think about some of the ways you can assist in better patient adherence and public safety regarding opioid use.

Case Study A

Mrs. Jones appears with a new prescription for hydrocodone, a pain medication, and states that she just left the doctor's office and that he told her to stop the medication she was previously on and start taking this one. She asks if it would be all right to give her brother the rest of her prescription because he doesn't have insurance and is on the same medication. Why would you tell her no, even though it is the same medication?

A prescription is written for a specific patient, and should never be taken by anyone other than that patient for whom it was prescribed. US Food and Drug Administration (FDA) regulations require that the label of any drug listed as a "controlled substance" in Schedules II, III, or IV of the Controlled Substance Act (CSA) must, when dispensed to or for a patient, contain the following warning: "CAUTION: Federal law prohibits the transfer of this drug to any person other than the patient for whom it was prescribed."

Encourage her to bring the remainder of her old pain medication in so that it can be disposed of properly. Explain that it is unsafe to leave it around the home, where it might be ingested by a child or someone might take it for abuse reasons. It could encourage a crime, or someone could take it by mistake.

Case Study B

As the advanced technician working in a busy community pharmacy, you must review the inventory for all Schedule II medications (CIIs) daily. When you check the log for all CIIs dispensed today, you notice a discrepancy of one fentanyl patch unaccounted for in the prescriptions. What would you do?

One of the options is to report this to the DEA's Rx Abuse Online Reporting program. It would be anonymous, and if you are worried about retribution or who might be involved, this would be an appropriate way to go. This could also be reported to your immediate supervisor, but regardless, it is important to report the incident. The loss to the store, the possible diversion, the possibility of one of your coworkers needing help with abuse, and the general public's safety all are reasons to get to the bottom of the situation.

ADVANCED TECHNICIAN OPPORTUNITIES IN CONTROLLED DRUG DIVERSION PREVENTION AND TRACKING PROGRAMS

There are many opportunities in the area of diversion monitoring, technology quality control, and loss prevention. Some of these involve reviewing pharmacy systems to look for patterns of abuse or detecting abnormalities within the system. Many of the state PDMPs are aligned with the patient's electronic health record (EHR), and this means that the series of events can be tracked from the computerized physician order entry (CPOE) to the administration of the medication at the patient's bedside.

Drug diversion can also occur prior to the transfer from the manufacturer to the intended dispensary. This type of diversion could be related to inventory control or even ordering practices. Loss-prevention specialists can look for patterns or discrepancies in what was ordered, what was received, and what was dispensed, all of which can be verified as part of a quality control program. Most automated storage and distribution systems have built-in reporting and safeguards to protect the user when removing medication, and these entries can be tracked to the second. Even pharmacies with manual record keeping use perpetual inventory methods. When a controlled substance is counted, it usually requires a second count, in addition to a record in a logbook of the starting amount and the current amount each time something is removed. The responsibilities of

these positions may involve staff training, investigation and gathering of facts for events, and process improvement initiatives based on data collected or audits conducted. There may also be challenges in working with outside agencies to promote awareness and provide current information if required for legal actions.

Some of the most important qualities needed for these positions include the following:
- Ability to distinguish between facts and probabilities when investigating incidents
- Ability to review data for patterns or to locate discrepancies
- Maintenance of current knowledge of local, state, and federal laws and regulations regarding controlled substances
- Ability to conduct audits and find possible risks, gaps in processes, or trends
- Good communication skills to work closely with others
- Ability to use automation/technology for tracking, auditing, and implementation of processes developed

Opioid abuse will continue to be a problem, and the development of better tracking and prevention and awareness programs will be a permanent focus of healthcare providers. Advanced technicians can play an important role in assisting pharmacy practice in better monitoring, improved reporting, and educating the public. Providing information at the first contact a patient has in the pharmacy and knowing the history of previous medication fills are of instrumental value to the profession. Recognizing signs of potential abuse, diversion, or patient nonadherence is key to medication safety and the future of a healthier society. Signs of abuse may include changes in someone's regular lifestyle routine, a sudden need for isolation, paranoia, or withdrawal. Abuse can affect work performance, decision making, appearance, and interactions with family. Sudden changes in daily patterns, such as coming in early or leaving late, can indicate secrecy or attempts at diversion. All technicians and other members of the pharmacy team should be conscious of the potential for abuse, and it is everyone's responsibility to look for signs of diversion and abuse and take the necessary steps to eliminate them.

REVIEW QUESTIONS

1. Which of the following could result in an opioid being prescribed for chronic pain?
   a. Postoperative pain
   b. Osteoarthritis
   c. Motor vehicle accident
   d. Both a and c
2. Which of the following best describes acute pain?
   a. Pain that lasts longer than 3 months
   b. Pain that lasts for at least 3 months
   c. Pain that heals before 3 months
   d. Both a and c

3. Which of the following opioids can be extracted from certain poppy plants?
   a. Fentanyl
   b. Morphine
   c. Heroin
   d. Cocaine
4. Which of the following is a synthetic opioid that can be 50 times more potent than morphine?
   a. Fentanyl
   b. Heroin
   c. Codeine
   d. Oxycodone
5. Which term describes taking more of a drug than what a physician has directed?
   a. Drug abuse
   b. Drug addiction
   c. Drug dependence
   d. Drug misuse
6. Which of the following, given via injection, can be used as a reversal for an opioid overdose if given in time?
   a. Naltrexone
   b. Naloxone
   c. Mechan
7. When a person has been taking an opioid and must increase the dose to maintain the same effects over time, it is referred to as which of the following?
   a. Drug addiction
   b. Drug dependence
   c. Drug tolerance
   d. Drug abuse

8. All of the following can be withdrawal symptoms EXCEPT:
   a. Agitation
   b. Depression
   c. Itching
   d. Sleepiness
9. Which of the following states had the fewest opioid prescriptions written in 2017?
   a. Vermont
   b. Hawaii
   c. Rhode Island
   d. Alabama
10. Which controlled substance electronic database program is operated in 49 states to date?
    a. PDMP
    b. MAT
    c. OUD
    d. HRPDMP

CRITICAL THINKING QUESTIONS

1. As an advanced pharmacy technician working in an MAT practice setting, how would you explain to a new technician what this means and what is provided for a patient?
2. How would you explain to patients the need to bring their unwanted medications to the store for destruction rather than leaving them in the cabinet, flushing them, or just throwing them in the trash at home?

REFERENCES

Lindsay, E. (2016). The High Cost of Drug Diversion. Retrieved December 26, 2019 from https://www.pharmacytimes.com/contributor/erica-lindsay-pharmd-mba-jd/2016/01/the-high-cost-of-drug-diversion.

Scholl, L., Seth, P., Kariisa, M., Wilson, N., & Baldwin, G. (December 21, 2018). Drug and Opioid-Involved Overdose Deaths–United States, 2013-2017. *WR Morb Mortal Wkly Rep*. ePub.

US Department of Health and Human Services. National Opioid Crisis. Retrieved December 27, 2019 from https://www.hhs.gov/opioids/.

Medication Verification

11

Learning Objectives

1. Discuss how the rising costs of medications are affecting pharmacy services.
2. Explain the advantages and major components of medication verification programs.
3. Explain the process of claims and reimbursement and the technology resources that are used to track medications and patients.
4. Discuss the advanced technician's role in improving patient medication adherence, improving efficiency, and reducing costs for the pharmacy.

Key Terms

Automated dispensing cabinet (ADC) Electronic cabinet used to dispense supplies or medications.

Automated dispensing devices (ADDs) Electronic devices used to dispense items such as medications or supplies.

Average sale price (ASP) Model for drug reimbursement pricing used by the Centers for Medicare and Medicaid Services (CMS).

Average wholesale price (AWP) Model for pricing of drug reimbursement used by insurance companies.

Barcode medication administration (BCMA) Tracking and dispensing system using the barcode found on products.

Billing Submission of a prescription to the pharmacy benefits manager (PBM) for payment, usually electronically.

Claim To file a request for payment.

Computerized physician order entry (CPOE) Process of electronic entry of physician orders.

Electronic health record (EHR) A patient's electronic record that includes health and medication information.

Electronic medication administration record (eMAR) Patient medication record that is kept electronically.

National Drug Code (NDC) unique 3-segment universal number identifying drug products

Pharmacy benefits manager (PBM) Controls the submission of claims and any payment to pharmacies as a representative of the insurance company.

Reimbursement Payment to a provider for services.

Shrinkage inventory loss due to theft or waste

INTRODUCTION

Today's pharmacy depends on the continuous flow of reimbursement, or payment for medications and clinical services provided. The daily operations of tracking, verification, and submission of claims must incorporate current technology to stay competitive (Fig. 11.1). As advanced technicians step into more critical roles, the medication verification systems that include dispensing and claims technology can be used to increase the clinical pharmacy services offered while pharmacists serve in more of a clinical role. Processes like medication, provider and payer verification, prior authorizations, and pricing accuracy can be monitored and better managed.

EFFECT OF COST OF MEDICATIONS ON TODAY'S PHARMACY SERVICES

The reimbursement from public payers such as third-party insurance has decreased over the years. Recently, the Centers for Medicare and Medicaid Services (CMS) also decreased its **average sale price (ASP)** margin from 6% to 4%. The ASP is determined by quarterly sales reported to Medicare. What does this mean? The reimbursement for a prescription is based on the ASP or **average wholesale price (AWP)** which is the cost of the medication plus vendor fees, the lower the percentage, the lower is the amount of reimbursement given to the pharmacy (Fig. 11.2). In addition, if a prescription is not billed correctly, or the patient or provider is incorrectly identified, there may be delays in payment for services or, in some cases, a forfeit of payment. Understanding the revenue cycle or **billing** process for a pharmacy is key to understanding how improvements can be made. Programs such as tech check tech (TCT) allow a pharmacy to use the expertise and training of advanced technicians and reduce the salary costs of additional pharmacists. To work properly, the system must contain accurate information, including correct medication, patient, price, and packaging information (see Chapter 5).

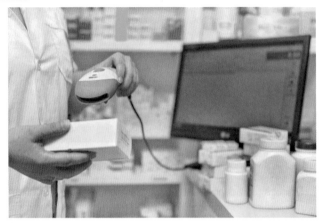

Fig. 11.1 Pharmacy tech using a barcode scanner for product verification. (Copyright @ iStock.com/MJ_Prototype.)

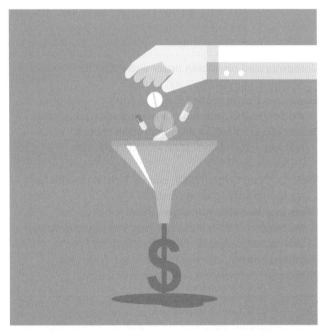

Fig. 11.2 Money for prescriptions. (Copyright @ iStock.com/Ja_inter.)

DATA WORKFLOW

Before the provider sends the prescription and the pharmacy fills it, there are several steps involved. Data entry must be performed, and verification of patient, payer, and medication must be incorporated into this process.

In community pharmacies this process includes verification of the patient using questions or validation of forms of identification. The insurance card should have name, social security number, and birthdate.

In an inpatient setting, such as hospital, this verification process may be a little different due to the patient conditions. Using an armband with registration information assigned at the time of admittance would be appropriate

The electronic system for third party claims is delivered through a process known as adjudication. The prescription is entered into the data base, and the claim is sent to a third party or Prescription Benefits Manager (PBM) who requests payment from the insurance listed in the patient's profile. If the insurance company pays, it sends through a co pay amount and PAID message. If it is rejected or not covered, it rejects and gives a coded message. This message may indicate drug is not on the formulary so not covered, or something is incorrect to match the patient to the insurance information. This occurs in a matter of seconds.

If the issue is with the drug that was entered for payment, such as the wrong NDC number, it could be rejected as well.

If the wrong **National Drug Code (NDC)** number is chosen, for example, the reimbursement can be different from what was actually dispensed. The pharmacy will be paid for the NDC entered into the system and not what was actually counted for the bottle. If the NDC number is obsolete and this isn't checked, the claim will be rejected as well. In addition, the "dispense as written" (DAW) code must be correct. The following is a list of codes typically used:

- DAW code 1: A substitution is *not* allowed by the physician.
- DAW code 2: Substitution allowed—patient requested that brand product be dispensed.
- DAW code 3: Substitution allowed—pharmacist selected product dispensed.
- DAW code 4: Substitution allowed—generic drug not in stock.

If the physician orders a "brand" drug specifically and it is not billed to the insurance accordingly, the correct reimbursement will be given for a lower generic drug rate, which means less money paid to the pharmacy.

One of the key tasks of the advanced technician is to ensure the claim is processed accurately and in a timely manner so that the pharmacy will receive payment promptly. If the demographic information for the patient, such as birthday, name, or address, does not match with the payer's information, this is not only a source for a potential medication error, but also the reimbursement may be rejected. This will cost additional time, which is money, and result in less profit for the pharmacy.

If the wrong payer is billed as a result of the wrong information being keyed during data entry, the claim will be rejected. This will also cause additional time and expense to the pharmacy's overall business.

INVENTORY MANAGEMENT

Ordering, receiving, stocking, and verifying medications kept in inventory are other important parts of medication verification. The use of technology, such as **barcode medication administration (BCMA)** or radiofrequency identification (RFID), or the medication's NDC number is typically used. The NDC number is a series of 10 digits to identify a medication. It contains three parts: labeler, product, and package. RFID numbers are used in warehouses to identify products, and the US Food and Drug Administration (FDA) now supports RFID use as a method of tracking products more efficiently. A unique number is assigned by the manufacturer, and any future transactions or movements of that product can be traced. The use of available technology over manual entry can eliminate common problems, such as unit of measure (UOM) errors. UOM errors involve a mistake in the units that are charged for and kept in inventory, such as vials of medication that contain 10 mL. If this was manually entered as vials of 1 mL by mistake, and pricing was based on a single unit being dispensed, the patient would be charged for 1 mL but receive 10 mL of medication, an additional 9 mL for free.

LINKING PURCHASING AND BILLING SYSTEMS

Some pharmacies, especially in large hospital systems, use different systems for purchasing and dispensing medications. The different systems must interface to ensure a consistent and accurate flow of information. This is where one of the verification systems, such as RFID, barcoding, and **automated dispensing devices (ADDs)**, can be used. The inventory is tracked from the supplier all the way through to the time when the patient's medication has been dispensed and is ready for electronic **claims** submission. Orders are entered through the **computerized physician order entry (CPOE)** system. The order is then systematically checked for adverse effects, drug interactions, and correct dosing regimens. Once this is complete, the medication can be linked to the **automated dispensing cabinet (ADC)** matching inventory and verified. Bedside verification scanning systems are used when administering medications in the hospital and include the person withdrawing the medication from the cabinet, the person administering the medication, and the patient receiving the dose. Not only is this best practice for patient safety and error prevention, but it also keeps revenue loss low. The five rights of medication administration can be incorporated into technology and a sophisticated tracking system. ADSs include tracking for users, expired drugs, overages, unused drugs, and other customized reporting the facility may need.

 Tech Note

In an evaluation of the impact of barcoding drugs in the pharmacy and checking them before they are sent to patient care units, one report noted that the dispensing error rate fell by 31% after barcode implementation in the pharmacy (Agrawal, 2009).

In community settings, the pharmacy management program tracks medication and patient information. The point-of-sale (POS) pharmacy system is the check system for the patient record of pickup and links compliance and adherence in the medication-dispensing process. This system allows the pharmacy to track available inventory, manage customers, securely accept payments, and incorporate e-prescribing. This system also allows prescriptions to be sent electronically to the pharmacy. This is also an important step in preventing errors and ensuring patient safety because it eliminates errors in the interpretation of handwriting, allows for faster turnaround, and aligns with the medication verification tracking system that uses today's available technology.

MANAGEMENT OF CURRENT STOCK

Shrinkage is an ever-present consideration in a pharmacy. Shrinkage includes inventory loss as a result of expiration, slow-moving medications, or errors. Suppliers coordinate automated replenishment methods through current technology and by tracking of medications that should be returned. Advanced technicians can perform routine reviews of these tracking tools to ensure medication inventory is appropriate for the facility. There should not be an excess of "slow movers," those drugs that aren't being dispensed regularly. Medications approaching expiration should be rotated to the front or returned for credit to the supplier if possible. If prescriptions are filled and dispensed in error, this can be very costly and a cause of preventable errors.

ERROR PREVENTION AND COMPLIANCE

Data-driven technology for reporting and compliance with regulations is an advantage of medication verification systems. Medication error reporting systems (MERSs) are in place in over 23 states, but many accrediting agencies, such as The Joint Commission, require reporting as well. The Institute for Safe Medicine Practices (ISMP) encourages reporting through the National Medication Errors Reporting Program (ISMP MERP). Information should be detailed and include the following (ISMP, 2019):

- The details of what went wrong or could go wrong
- The causes and contributing factors of the event
- How the event or condition was discovered or intercepted
- The actual or potential outcome of the involved patient(s)
- Recommendations for error prevention
- Product names, dosage forms, and dose/strength (For product-specific concerns [e.g., labeling and packaging risks], the manufacturer should be included.)
- Specific information regarding the model, build, and manufacturer of involved healthcare information technology and medication-related devices
- Any associated materials that help support the report being submitted (e.g., images of devices, display screens, products, containers, labels, de-identified prescription orders)

If a patient experiences an adverse drug effect (ADE), this can also be reported within the facility's medication verification system for record-keeping purposes. For example, errors can be manually entered and then added to a statistical software program for analysis. The use of these data when performing quality control provides accurate details along with corresponding information that can be used to prevent future errors.

 Tech Note

Did you know medication errors can include near misses and close calls?

Case Study

A technician is working in the anticoagulant clinic of a hospital. As the medication reconciliation technician, she must record the history of the patient's medications before the patient is moved to a room on the floor. While reviewing the records in the system, she notices there had been a previous "near miss" reported within the facility's documentation of the patient concerning a dose of warfarin administered from an ADC during an earlier stay.

Should this be brought to the attention of the pharmacist, and if so, what type of information would be helpful in researching the incident?

The reporting of a near miss is very important and should be reviewed immediately. Reasons as to why, whom, when, what the circumstances were, and any other important information should be reviewed. What if the ADC has the incorrect dose or medication loaded in a pocket? Had the administering personnel had other incidents? Was the order been entered correctly? Was the medication verified by BCMA, RFID, or NDC? Did any follow-up occur after the report?

PATIENT ADHERENCE IMPROVEMENT

The use of electronic medication verification programs also improves medication adherence. The link to the patient's **electronic health record (EHR)** and **electronic medication administration record (eMAR)** also provides a real-time record and checkpoint that can be shared by many healthcare professionals involved in the patient's adherence plan. The verification process of medications, patients, and payer sources should be integral parts of providing medications and services to the patient (Fig. 11.3).

Pharmacy billing information is part of the medication reconciliation process and should include any patient assistance for medications if needed. As discussed previously, there are many reasons for patients not adhering to a medication regimen. Cost is certainly a concern, and medications are prescribed every day that patients cannot afford. By reviewing accurate medication verification information, the advanced technician can assist the patient in locating resources that may be available. An alert in the system when performing data entry may indicate that the manufacturer offers reduced costs, coupons, or discounts.

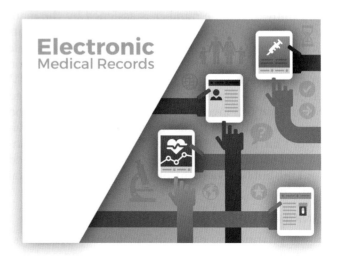

Fig. 11.3 Example of an electronic health record (EHR). (Copyright @ iStock.com/filo.)

In addition, there are built-in systems that accept refill requests and provide reminder alerts for refills in some systems. Medication synchronization (see Chapter 8) is designed to align the patient's medications so that they are due at the same time each month. An automatic refill program can also alert the pharmacist to patients who are not regularly picking up their scheduled medications. Once this information is reviewed, an intervention can occur to try to get the patient back to adherence.

ADVANCED TECHNICIAN ROLES IN MEDICATION VERIFICATION

Medication must be delivered at the right cost for pharmacies to survive in today's healthcare environment. With a lean, quality-driven approach, pharmacies must be proactive and weigh the cost of advanced technology with medication verification against positive patient outcomes and safety. They must use the staff to the fullest potential, and advanced technicians can assist in this endeavor.

Some common tasks associated with medication verification technician roles include the following:
- Managing user databases and updates to new employees and deleting inactive users to maintain a current record of users in the system for tracking purposes
- Setting up, installing, and troubleshooting problems with the verification system
- Ensuring any formulary changes have been implemented, including NDCs, barcodes, or RFID tags as applicable
- Removing waste and excess medications to reduce shrinkage and prevent errors
- Reporting of errors or ADEs to agencies or organizations as required
- Establishing training for personnel on system requirements and participating in a TCT program if applicable

- Establishing and maintaining reports as the facility requires (out of stock, expires, discrepancies, errors)
- Incorporating reporting information into quality assurance (QA) and quality control (QC) programs
- Monitoring systems communication for alignment of information
- Interacting with outside suppliers and payer sources to align correct reimbursement and billing processes
- Interacting directly with patients for medication assistance, refill reminders, synchronization, and other tools to promote adherence

When advanced technicians are involved in the day-to-day activity of medication verification with the use of technology, the pharmacist is afforded more time with patients and has the ability to expand the services offered to patients. Realigning duties and streamlining processes will allow the pharmacy to continue to optimize efficiency and promote the best care at the best value for patients.

REVIEW QUESTIONS

1. Which of the following is NOT a feature of an electronic medication verification program?
   a. Increases staffing
   b. Prevents errors
   c. Increases shrinkage
   d. Reduces shrinkage
2. Which of the following is an electronic means of identification for medication verification?
   a. BCMA
   b. RFID
   c. NDC
   d. All of the above
3. Which of the following describes the system used to enter orders from the physician?
   a. RFID
   b. NDC
   c. CPOE
   d. BCMA
4. Which abbreviation describes the physician's wishes for a specific brand of medication to be prescribed?
   a. DAW
   b. DRW
   c. NAW
   d. NDC

5. Which term describes the method the CMS uses to determine costs for reimbursement for medications?
   a. AWP
   b. ASP
   c. ADS
   d. ADC
6. Which of the following is the abbreviation for how a third-party (insurance) provider would calculate reimbursement for a drug?
   a. AWP
   b. ASP
   c. ADC
   d. ADS
7. All of the following are common duties a medication verification technician might perform EXCEPT:
   a. Facilitate setup
   b. Report error to ISMP
   c. Adjust doses
   d. Adjust pricing of drug
8. Which term best describes the alignment of a patient's medication refills on the same day each month?
   a. Synchronization
   b. Medication adherence
   c. Medication reconciliation
   d. Automatic refill reminders
9. If a patient experiences an unwanted side effect from a medication, what is the term used?
   a. ADC
   b. ADE
   c. ADS
   d. ASP
10. If a patient is dispensed a vial of 10 mL of insulin and the charge in the system is for 1 mL, what type of error is this?
    a. UOM
    b. ASP
    c. AWP
    d. DAW

CRITICAL THINKING QUESTIONS

1. As a pharmacy medication assistance technician, you are responsible for monitoring the automatic refill program and notice that Ms. Jones never picked up a prescription that was written last month, and it was put on hold. What type of assistance could you offer?
2. Discuss the advantages of an electronic means, such as RFID, for the tracking of medications through a system.

REFERENCES

Agrawal, A. (2009). Medication errors: prevention using information technology systems. *British journal of clinical pharmacology*, 67(6), 681–686. https://doi.org/10.1111/j.1365-2125.2009.03427.x.

Institute for Safe Medication Practices. Report a Medication Error. Retrieved December 11, 2019 from https://www.ismp.org/report-error/merp.

12 Education and Training

Learning Objectives

1. Discuss advanced certifications and certificates available for pharmacy technicians.
2. Review the outline and content of certified compounded sterile preparation technician (CSPT) certification and the certificates being offered to today's technicians who wish

to become a certified pharmacy technician advanced (CPhT-Adv).
3. Discuss the education and training required for technicians to advance their careers and serve in advanced technician roles.

Key Term

Certified compounded sterile preparation technician (CSPT) Certification offered by the Pharmacy Technician Certification Board (PTCB) in sterile compounding for technicians.

INTRODUCTION

The role of pharmacy technicians is rapidly changing, and requirements for education and training are necessary for patient safety (Fig. 12.1). With the advances in medicine and treatments and the shift toward a patient-centered model, the profession requires that pharmacists perform a more clinical role. Tasks such as dispensing, compounding, and managing inventory, which were once solely for pharmacists, are now being performed by technicians. Organizations such as the American Society of Health-System Pharmacists (ASHP) and the Pharmacy Technician Certification Board (PTCB) have led the way to empower technicians by promoting regulations. The PTCB began offering specialty certificates in 2019, with more on the horizon. This has expanded technician responsibilities and allows technicians to play a much bigger role in optimal patient care practices.

PHARMACY TECHNICIAN CERTIFICATION BOARD

Currently, 21 states require technicians to be certified to work in the state (PTCB, 2019). In the past, on-the-job training was the most common way technicians were trained. Obtaining an education through an accredited program or a PTCB-approved program and then becoming a certified pharmacy technician (CPhT) through the PTCB examination process is the preferred method today. Once working as a technician, there are

opportunities to advance your skills through work experience, specialty exams, and training. Currently, the PTCB offers an advanced specialty certification and two certificates, with additional certifications planned for the future.

CERTIFIED COMPOUNDED STERILE PREPARATION TECHNICIAN CERTIFICATION

The PTCB offers an advanced certification in sterile compounding, the **certified compounded sterile preparation technician (CSPT)**. In order to take the exam, one must be a CPhT and either have completed a PTCB-recognized program and have 1 year of experience in sterile compounding *or* have 3 years of continuous work experience in sterile compounding. The exam is multiple choice and covers hazardous and nonhazardous products. The areas covered are listed in Table 12.1.

The exam covers the main aspects associated with sterile compounding, and the following list provides a description of the types of questions that are covered: Medications and Components

- Pharmacology of drugs, including names, classes, side effects, dosing, and indications for use
- Information associated with compounds, including Safety Data Sheets (SDSs), patient information, and references
- Storage, compatibility, and factors affecting stability

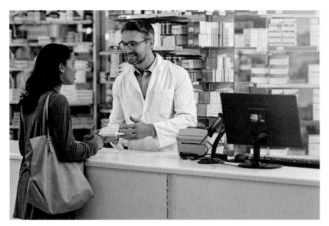

Fig. 12.1 Pharmacy technician talking with a patient. (Copyright @ Grady Reese/Getty Images.)

Facilities and Equipment
- Types of primary engineering controls (laminar airflow workspace [LAFW], biological safety cabinet [BSC], compounding aseptic containment isolator [CACI]) and proper use
- Types of secondary engineering controls (areas or rooms, e.g., anteroom or buffer room)
- Monitoring of environment, such as temperature and humidity
- Sampling for both primary and secondary controls

Procedures
- Personnel training and competency requirements
- Handwashing, personal hygiene, and garbing
- Aseptic technique using sterile and nonsterile ingredients

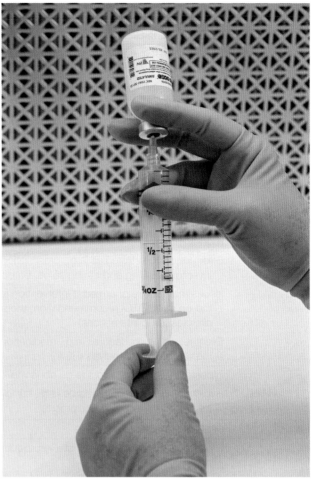

Fig. 12.2 Technician withdrawing contents from a vial. (From Davis, K., & Guerra, A. [2019]. *Mosby's pharmacy technician* [5th ed.]. St. Louis, MO: Elsevier.)

Table **12.1**	Pharmacy Technician Certification Exam (PTCE) Content Outline	
Knowledge domains and areas	**Percentage of PTCE exam content**	
1.	**MEDICATIONS**	**40%**
1.1	Generic names, brand names, and classifications of medications	
1.2	Therapeutic equivalence	
1.3	Common and life-threatening drug interactions and contraindications (e.g., drug–disease, drug–drug, drug–dietary supplement, drug–laboratory, drug–nutrient)	
1.4	Strengths/dose, dosage forms, routes of administration, special handling and administration instructions, and duration of drug therapy	
1.5	Common and severe medication side effects, adverse effects, and allergies	
1.6	Indications of medications and dietary supplements	
1.7*	Drug stability (e.g., oral suspensions, insulin, reconstitutables, injectables, vaccinations)	
1.8	Narrow therapeutic index (NTI) medications	
1.9	Physical and chemical incompatibilities related to nonsterile compounding and reconstitution	
1.10	Proper storage of medications (e.g., temperature ranges, light sensitivity, restricted access)	

Continued

Table 12.1	Pharmacy Technician Certification Exam (PTCE) Content Outline—cont'd		
2.	**FEDERAL REQUIREMENTS**	**12.5%**	
2.1	Federal requirements for handling and disposal of nonhazardous, hazardous, and pharmaceutical substances and waste		
2.2*	Federal requirements for controlled substance prescriptions (i.e., new, refill, transfer) and US Drug Enforcement Agency (DEA) controlled substance schedules		
2.3	Federal requirements (e.g., DEA, US Food and Drug Administration [FDA]) for controlled substances, i.e., receiving, storing, ordering, labeling, dispensing, reverse distribution, take-back programs, and loss or theft of)		
2.4*	Federal requirements for restricted drug programs and related medication processing (e.g., pseudoephedrine, risk evaluation and mitigation strategies [REMS])		
2.5	FDA recall requirements (e.g., medications, devices, supplies, supplements, classifications)		
3.	**PATIENT SAFETY AND QUALITY ASSURANCE**	**26.25%**	
3.1	High-alert/high-risk medications and look-alike/sound-alike (LASA) medications		
3.2	Error prevention strategies (e.g., prescription or medication order to correct patient, Tall Man lettering, separating inventory, leading and trailing zeros, barcode usage, limit use of error-prone abbreviations)		
3.3*	Issues that require pharmacist intervention (e.g., drug utilization review [DUR], adverse drug event [ADE], over-the-counter [OTC] recommendation, therapeutic substitution, misuse, adherence, postimmunization follow-up, allergies, drug interactions)		
3.4	Event reporting procedures (e.g., medication errors, adverse effects, and product integrity, MedWatch, near miss, root-cause analysis [RCA])		
3.5*	Types of prescription errors (e.g., abnormal doses, early refill, incorrect quantity, incorrect patient, incorrect drug)		
3.6	Hygiene and cleaning standards (e.g., handwashing; personal protective equipment [PPE]; cleaning counting trays, countertop, and equipment)		
4.	**ORDER ENTRY AND PROCESSING**	**21.25%**	
4.1*	Procedures to compound nonsterile products (e.g., ointments, mixtures, liquids, emulsions, suppositories, enemas)		
4.2*	Formulas, calculations, ratios, proportions, alligations, conversions, Sig codes (e.g., b.i.d.k, t.i.d., Roman numerals), abbreviations, medical terminology, and symbols for days' supply, quantity, dose, concentration, dilutions		
4.3*	Equipment/supplies required for drug administration (e.g., package size, unit dose, diabetic supplies, spacers, oral and injectable syringes)		
4.4*	Lot numbers, expiration dates, and National Drug Code (NDC) numbers		
4.5	Procedures for identifying and returning dispensable, nondispensable, and expired medications and supplies (e.g., credit return, return to stock, reverse distribution)		

Reprinted with permission from the Pharmacy Technician Certification Board (PTCB).

- Cleaning and disinfecting procedures of primary and secondary equipment/facilities
- Safety and disposal
- Calculations used in compounding
- Compounding total parenteral nutrition (TPN) solutions, including weighing volumetrically
- Record keeping and documentation
Handling, packaging, and storage
- Proper packaging, handling, and storage for hazardous and nonhazardous compounds
- Types of containers and packaging used

There is also a listing of compounding-related medications that are included as part of the material covered in the exam. This information can be found at https://www.ptcb.org/credentials/certified-compounded-sterile-preparation-technician.

CERTIFIED PHARMACY TECHNICIAN ADVANCED

In addition to the sterile compounding certification, the PTCB began offering a set of advanced certificates to gain a credential of certified pharmacy technician advanced (CPhT-Adv). To date, these are certificate programs related to medication history and product verification, with others coming soon. Completing at least four of the five certificates *or* three certificates and the sterile compounding certification is required for the CPhT-Adv. These exams are multiple choice and in line with the 2-hour limit, similar to the CPhT exam.

PTCB MEDICATION HISTORY CERTIFICATE

The content for the medication history certificate relates to taking patient histories and patient safety and

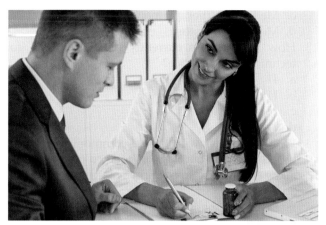

Fig. 12.3 Technician completing a medication history for a new patient. (Copyright © iStock.com/megaflopp.)

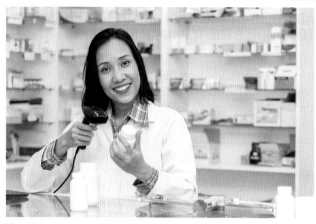

Fig. 12.4 Pharmacy technician scanning a bottle of medication using a barcode reader. (Copyright © iStock.com/AvigatorPhotographer.)

quality assurance (Fig. 12.3). The content is broken into two sections, with 45% covering concepts and terminology and 55% covering patient safety. (For more information to aid with this certificate, refer to Chapters 7 and 8). The general outline of the exam includes the following:

- Patient adherence concepts and terminology, such as *intolerance* and *allergies*
- Vaccines and scheduling
- Use of appropriate medical terminology for both patients and caregivers
- Impact of medication errors and prevention techniques
- Interpretation of prescriptions, including dosing, directions, and route of administration
- Health Insurance Portability and Accountability Act (HIPAA) regulations and ways to communicate with patients
- Use of medication aids, such as pillboxes and calendars
- Patient identifier procedures
- Assistance with patient reporting of medication history and ways to stay on dosing schedule

PTCB TECHNICIAN PRODUCT VERIFICATION CERTIFICATE

The exam for the technician product verification (TPV) certificate has 120 multiple-choice questions that provide a prescription or order label to align with images of the product for verification. The concepts covered include the following:

- Identifying correct name, strength, and dosage form of the medication
- Correct calculations for the days' supply and amount to be dispensed
- Verification of product information, such as expiration date, lot numbers, or other identifiers

For more information regarding related content, refer to Chapter 11 (Fig. 12.4).

ADDITIONAL PTCB CERTIFICATES UNDER DEVELOPMENT

The additional certificates under development by the PTCB include three other exams by which advanced technicians can demonstrate competencies for the achievement of the CPhT-Adv. These include the following:

- Controlled substances and diversion (see Chapter 10 for related content)
- Billing and reimbursement (see Chapter 6 for related content)
- Hazardous drugs (see Chapter 9 for related content)

 Tech Note

The PTCB has created digital badges to display the accomplishment of each of the certificates offered to date (Fig. 12.5).

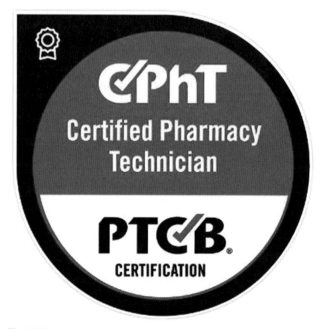

Fig. 12.5 Sample digital badge for a technician certified by the Pharmacy Technician Certification Board (PTCB). (Courtesy Pharmacy Technician Certification Board, Washington, D.C.)

ADDITIONAL EDUCATION AND OPPORTUNITIES TO ADVANCE THE TECHNICIAN'S CAREER

There are many courses and continuing education programs provided by large organizations, employers, and private providers that are accredited by the Accreditation Council for Pharmacy Education (ACPE). These courses are often online and provide credit for maintaining CPhT status.

There are also hands-on courses offered by national and state organizations in a variety of subject areas. The Society for the Education of Pharmacy Technicians (SEPhT, 2020) offers boot camps in several areas that include live training: sterile and nonsterile compounding certificates with 12 hours of continuing education units (CEUs), medication management therapy, inventory and repackaging (using automated dispensing cabinet), emergency and disaster planning, and wellness clinic with disease prevention. The National Pharmacy Technician Association (NPTA, n.d.) offers certificates in sterile products, hazardous products, and compounding. Critical Point IV (2020) offers live skills camps in sterile compounding and e-learning courses and webinars.

There are several providers of continuing education. Power-Pak C.E. (2020) offers a certificate in medication management therapy. The ASHP has offerings for continued education as well through the PharmacyTechCE program (ASHP, 2020).

As a practicing pharmacy technician, it is always best to stay current in the practice and seek out information that will expand your knowledge base and advance your career. Participating in pharmacy meetings at the local and state levels is also a good resource for gaining experience and making connections within the profession. Completing online courses through colleges or companies that provide continuing education is often affordable and will also provide additional knowledge. Many employers will reimburse or cover training if requested.

Never stand still! There is always more to learn, and opportunities for technicians who wish to advance their careers will continue to grow.

REVIEW QUESTIONS

1. Which of the following is NOT one of the PTCB certificates *currently* offered for the advanced CPhT?
   a. CPhT
   b. Medication history
   c. Product verification
   d. Billing and reimbursement
2. Critical Point offers which of the following related courses?
   a. Nonsterile compounding
   b. Sterile compounding
   c. Medication therapy management
   d. Medication history
3. How many states currently require a CPhT for technicians to practice?
   a. 41
   b. 11
   c. 28
   d. 21
4. Which of the following tasks is commonly performed by advanced technicians in today's pharmacies to allow pharmacists to perform a more clinical role?
   a. Dispensing
   b. Inventory management
   c. Compounding
   d. Counseling
5. Which of the following areas covers over 50% of the content for the CSPT certification?
   a. Sterile procedures
   b. Handling and packaging
   c. Facilities and equipment
   d. Medications
6. What is PTCB's advanced credential once a certified technician has completed the 4 of 5 advanced certificates offered by the organization?
   a. CPhT
   b. CPhT-Adv
   c. ADV-CPhT
   d. CSPT-Adv
7. All of the following are types of primary engineering controls for sterile compounding EXCEPT:
   a. LAFW
   b. Anteroom
   c. BSC
   d. CACI
8. The content for which certificate exam is broken into two sections, with 45% covering concepts and terminology and 55% for patient safety?
   a. CPhT
   b. CPhT-Adv
   c. Product verification
   d. Medication history
9. Which of the following is a pathway for a CPhT to achieve the CPhT-Adv designation?
   a. Completing four of the five PTCB certificates
   b. Completing three PTCB certificates and the CSPT certification
   c. Completing five PTCB certificates
   d. Both a and b
10. How many years of continuous experience in sterile compounding are required to be eligible to take the CSPT exam without completing a PTCB-recognized program?
    a. 2 years
    b. 1 year
    c. 5 years
    d. 3 years

CRITICAL THINKING QUESTION

1. As a new graduate and recently hired CPhT in a hospital, what would be the best way to advance your career in the area of medication reconciliation, other than completing the PTCB medication history certificate?

REFERENCES

American Society of Health-System Pharmacists. (2020). *PharmacyTechCE*. Retrieved January 2, 2020 from https://www.ashp.org/Pharmacy-Technician/About-Pharmacy-Technicians/Pharmacy-Technician-Development/PharmacyTech-CE.

Critical Point IV. (2020). *View our Training Dates*. Retrieved Jan 2, 2020 from https://www.criticalpoint.info/.

National Pharmacy Technician Organization. (n.d.). Certificate Programs. Retrieved Jan 2, 2020 from http://www.pharmacytechnician.org/en/cms/?452.

Pharmacy Technician Certification Board. (2019). https://www.ptcb.org/resources/state-regulations-and-map.

Power-Pak, C. E. (2020). *MTM Program for Pharmacy Technicians*. Retrieved December 30, 2019 from https://www.powerpak.com/mtmpht10/.

Society for Education of Pharmacy Technicians. (2020). *Offers ACPE Skills Camps and Certifications*. Retrieved Jan 1, 2020 from http://thesepht.org/index.php?option=com_content&view=featured&Itemid=136.

Appendix

1. Which of the following organizations accredits continuing education for certified technicians?
   a. ACPE
   b. ASHP
   c. PTCB
   d. NHA
2. Which of the following describes the process of achieving a certain level of achievement through the completion of a competency-based exam?
   a. Certification
   b. Licensure
   c. Registration
   d. All of the above
3. What percentage of adult Americans are said to have a chronic illness?
   a. 30%
   b. 40%
   c. 50%
   d. 60%
4. Which of the following terms describes a collaboration of The Joint Commission with other healthcare providers to provide patient-centered care?
   a. POCT
   b. PCPP
   c. PODS
   d. PTCT
5. Point-of-care testing (POCT) includes which of the following elements designed to enhance the overall well-being of the patient?
   a. Smoking cessation
   b. Diet education
   c. Cholesterol screening
   d. All of the above
6. Key points from the Pharmacy Technician Certification Board (PTCB) stakeholder conference include all of the following EXCEPT:
   a. State requirement variability
   b. Compensation for trained technicians
   c. Certification requirements
   d. Entry-level requirements
7. Clinically oriented pharmacy technicians can provide support and expertise in which of the following areas?
   a. Determining disease outcomes
   b. Monitoring lab results
   c. Tracking medication errors
   d. Both b and c

8. An advanced technician can participate in the patient-centered care approach by assisting in which of the following?
   a. Recording lab results
   b. Collecting a patient's medication history
   c. Sharing medication information with nurses and other staff
   d. All of the above
9. Reviewing a patient's medication history allows a pharmacy to do all of the following EXCEPT:
   a. Identify adherence issues
   b. Identify untimely fills or refills
   c. Prevent future medication
   d. Identify choice of insurance coverage
10. All of the following additional services can be performed in today's pharmacy by advanced technicians EXCEPT:
    a. Immunizations
    b. Collecting medication histories
    c. Point-of-care testing
    d. Therapeutic counseling for wellness and disease prevention
11. Rewards for advanced technicians who demonstrate good leadership skills usually include all of the following EXCEPT:
    a. Job satisfaction
    b. Recognition
    c. Better work hours
    d. Advancement to other positions
12. Which of the following terms describes value-based care?
    a. Fee for care
    b. Accountable care
    c. Affordable care
    d. Appropriate care
13. All of the following are goals of an interdisciplinary care team for the patient EXCEPT:
    a. Management of physical needs
    b. Management of psychological needs
    c. Management of financial needs
    d. Management of spiritual needs
14. Tools for the management of disease commonly used by the primary care provider include which of the following?
    a. Surgery
    b. Diagnostic tests
    c. Medications
    d. All of the above

15. Which of the following organizations focuses on healthcare through the creation of National Patient Safety Goals?
    a. ASHP
    b. PTCB
    c. The Joint Commission
    d. ICT

16. Advantages of the use of decentralized pharmacies include all of the following EXCEPT:
    a. Less delay in administration of services
    b. Specialty trained personnel performing tasks
    c. Direct channel of communication among providers
    d. Higher reimbursement for services as a result of insurance incentives

17. According to the Practice Advancement Initiative (PAI) model, to allow more time for pharmacists to participate in direct patient care, which of the following roles should an advanced technician be used in?
    a. Performance of traditional preparation of medications
    b. Performance of distribution of medications
    c. Performance of advanced responsibilities
    d. All of the above

18. How does the use of proper workspace placement increase efficiency in pharmacy distribution?
    a. Reduces the number of steps required for a task
    b. Allows for fewer technicians to be hired
    c. Allows for less shelving to be needed
    d. Reduces amount of inventory needed

19. Which of the following is the main goal of the patient-centered model?
    a. Lower cost for medications
    b. Improved patient outcomes
    c. Fewer medications prescribed
    d. Employer incentives

20. Why would an employee survey ask the question, "How many hours do you sleep a night?"
    a. May indicate high stress levels
    b. May indicate insomnia is present
    c. May indicate sleep apnea is present
    d. All of the above

21. When indicating the maximum inventory replenishment amount to be kept in an automated dispensing cabinet (ADC), what term is used to identify the amount?
    a. PAR
    b. BPOE
    c. NDC
    d. RFID

22. What is the term used to describe the electronic record of medication administration for a patient?
    a. EHR
    b. eMAR
    c. eSCRIPT
    d. CPOE

23. What term is used to describe research that investigates how one's DNA is related to different drug actions?
    a. Pharmacokinetics
    b. Pharmacogenetics
    c. Pharmacology
    d. Pharmacokinetics

24. What is the term used to describe the process of using predetermined guidelines for a patient's care provided by a physician?
    a. Policies
    b. Procedures
    c. eSCRIPT
    d. Protocol

25. Which of the following would be considered durable medical equipment?
    a. Wheelchair
    b. Insulin syringes
    c. Wound care dressing
    d. Inhaler

26. What is the term used to describe medications being prepared for once-a-month pickup in special packaging known as "unit of use"?
    a. Synchronization
    b. Automatic fill
    c. Medication reconciliation
    d. Medication management

27. When preparing a medication reconciliation report, which of the following is required to be recorded?
    a. Prescriptions
    b. Over-the-counter supplements
    c. Vitamins
    d. All of the above

28. Which of the following conditions applies to a patient with chronic obstructive pulmonary disease (COPD) who requires ongoing medication and treatment?
    a. Acute condition
    b. Continuous condition
    c. Chronic condition
    d. None of the above

29. Which of the following conditions applies to a patient who has pneumonia and requires medication?
    a. Acute condition
    b. Continuous condition
    c. Chronic condition
    d. None of the above

30. Which of the following medications would be LEAST associated with nonpersistence for some patients?
    a. Antibiotic medication
    b. Diabetes medication
    c. High blood pressure medication
    d. Pain medication

31. Which of the following might occur if a patient is displaying nonfulfillment adherence after a primary provider appointment for an acute respiratory condition?

a. Patient seeks a second opinion.
b. Patient buys an over-the-counter cough/cold product.
c. Patient picks up a prescription.
d. Patient seeks advice of a pharmacist.

32. Which of the following describes a patient skipping doses or realigning times for administration to suit a daily schedule?
a. Nonconforming adherence
b. Nonpersistence adherence
c. Nonfulfillment adherence
d. None of the above

33. Some of the reasons that patients do not adhere to medication regimens include all of the following EXCEPT:
a. Employer incentives
b. Cost
c. Access
d. Dosing schedule

34. As an advanced technician working in a busy retail setting, which of the following would be most appropriate to assist a person who routinely misses monthly prescription fill dates?
a. Offering a pillbox
b. Offering medication synchronization services
c. Offering counseling
d. Offering non–child-proof lids

35. What is the term used to describe the testing method to determine the presence of microorganisms on the hands?
a. Gloved fingertip sampling
b. Surface sampling
c. Media fill testing
d. Aseptic technique observation

36. What is the term used to describe the testing method to determine a compounder's aseptic technique from a compounded sterile preparation (CSP)?
a. Media fill testing
b. Gloved fingertip testing
c. Surface sampling
d. Handwashing observation

37. Medications considered hazardous (not chemotherapy) should be disposed of a container of which color?
a. Yellow
b. Black
c. Red
d. Blue

38. The containment primary engineering control (C-PEC) most commonly used for the preparation of a hazardous drug compounded sterile preparation (CSP) is which of the following?
a. BSC
b. LAFW
c. LAFS
d. Isolator

39. To find out if a drug is considered hazardous, which of the following resources would be most appropriate for a current listing?
a. NIOSH
b. ASHP
c. *United States Pharmacopeia* chapter 797
d. *United States Pharmacopeia* chapter 800

40. Withdrawing a hazardous drug from a vial requires the use of which of the following special devices?
a. Vented needle
b. Filter needle
c. CSTD
d. C-PEC

41. A state board of pharmacy inspector visiting a compounding facility will ask for all of the following items EXCEPT:
a. Cleaning logs
b. Media fill results
c. Temperature log for refrigerator
d. Salary of compounding personnel

42. If you have completed the sterile compounding certification from the Pharmacy Technician Certification Board (PTCB), what designation would you have?
a. CPhT
b. CSPT
c. CPhT-Adv
d. ADV-CSPT

43. What is the term used to identify the record of a patient's compounded sterile preparation (CSP) directions, storage, and ingredients information?
a. CR
b. MFR
c. SOP
d. Prescription

44. Which term describes compounded sterile preparations (CSPs) assigned a beyond-use date (BUD) of less than 12 hours at room temperature or 24 hours or less if refrigerated?
a. Category 1
b. Category 2
c. Category 3
d. Category 4

45. Which term describes compounded sterile preparations (CSPs) assigned a beyond-use date (BUD) of more than 12 hours at room temperature or 24 hours or greater if refrigerated?
a. Category 1
b. Category 2
c. Category 3
d. Category 4

46. All of the following are considered compounded sterile preparations (CSPs) EXCEPT:
a. Otic preparations
b. Ophthalmic preparations
c. Bronchial inhalations
d. Cavity irrigations

47. Pain symptoms from an injury lasting 2 weeks would be best described as which of the following types of conditions?
    a. Acute pain
    b. Chronic pain
    c. Moderate pain
    d. Severe pain

48. What is the name of the electronic tracking program offered in many states that aims to curb the abuse of controlled substances?
    a. PDMP
    b. EHR
    c. CPOE
    d. RXabuse

49. All of the following would be commonly included in the medication-assisted treatment used to treat heroin addiction EXCEPT:
    a. Counseling
    b. Therapy
    c. Use of methadone
    d. Use of naloxone

50. Which of the following consequences to society are often seen as a result of the opioid crisis?
    a. Loss of work time
    b. Higher crime rates
    c. Higher vehicle insurance premiums
    d. All of the above

51. All of the following are considered opiates EXCEPT:
    a. Heroin
    b. Morphine
    c. Codeine
    d. Fentanyl

52. Which of the following terms describes the payment for services from a provider?
    a. Claim submission
    b. Reimbursement
    c. Incentive
    d. Billing

53. Which term describes the pharmacy code used when a generic drug is not in stock and a substitution is allowed?
    a. DAW1
    b. DAW2
    c. DAW3
    d. DAW4

54. What code would be used if a patient refused a generic substitution and insisted on the brand of the drug to be filled?
    a. DAW1
    b. DAW2

    c. DAW3
    d. DAW4

55. When reporting a medication error to the National Medication Errors Reporting Program (MERP), all of the following are recommended to be included EXCEPT:
    a. Outcome (results) to patient
    b. Cause of error
    c. Recommendations for prevention
    d. Demographic information for patient

56. Which of the following is currently offered as a specialty compounding certification from the Pharmacy Technician Certification Board (PTCB)?
    a. Medication history
    b. Product verification
    c. CPhT
    d. CSPT

57. The medication history certificate offered by the Pharmacy Technician Certification Board (PTCB) is broken into which of the following categories?
    a. Terminology and safety
    b. Dispensing and safety
    c. Medications and error prevention
    d. Compounding and safety

58. Which of the following specialty certificates is dedicated to the knowledge of calculations, dosage forms, and brand and generic names of drugs?
    a. TPV
    b. CSPT
    c. CPhT
    d. Adv-CPhT

59. Which specialty certification requires an understanding of TPN compounding techniques?
    a. CSPT
    b. TPV
    c. CPhT
    d. Adv-CPhT

60. Which of the specialty certificates required knowledge of vaccines and scheduling?
    a. CSPT
    b. CPhT
    c. TPV
    d. Medication history

Glossary

Accreditation Council for Pharmacy Education (ACPE) An organization that provides continuing education (CE) for pharmacy practitioners.

Acute condition An abrupt onset of a disease or condition.

Acute pain Pain that usually starts suddenly and last less than 3 months.

American Society of Health-System Pharmacists (ASHP) Organization whose mission is to support pharmacy professionals and promote patient medication safety.

Analytics The discovery, interpretation, and communication of meaningful patterns in data.

Aseptic technique Procedures used to prevent contamination of compounded sterile preparations (CSPs).

ASHP/ACPE A collaboration between the American Society of Health-System Pharmacists (ASHP) and the Accreditation Council for Pharmacy Education (ACPE) for accrediting technician training courses.

Automated dispensing cabinet (ADC) Electronic cabinet used to dispense supplies or medications.

Automated dispensing devices (ADDs) Electronic devices used to dispense items such as medications or supplies.

Average sale price (ASP) Model for drug reimbursement pricing used by the Centers for Medicare and Medicaid Services (CMS).

Average wholesale price (AWP) Model for pricing of drug reimbursement used by insurance companies.

Barcode medication administration (BCMA) Tracking and dispensing system that uses the barcodes found on products.

Beyond-use date (BUD) Date assigned at time of compounding, after which date the product should no longer be used and should be discarded.

Billing Submission of a prescription to the pharmacy benefits manager (PBM) for payment, usually electronically.

Board of pharmacy (BOP) State agency responsible for licensing, registration, or regulating the responsibilities of pharmacists and technicians.

Career ladder System using experience and knowledge to determine levels of responsibilities.

Certification Indicates successful completion of a certain level of achievement through passing a competency-based exam.

Certified compounded sterile preparation technician (CSPT) Certification offered by the Pharmacy Technician Certification Board (PTCB) in sterile compounding for technicians.

Certified pharmacy technician (CPhT) A technician who has successfully passed the national certification exam.

Chronic condition A condition that persists for longer than 3 months and is ongoing.

Chronic pain Pain, usually caused by a condition or disease, that lasts more than 3 months.

Claim To file a request for payment.

Comorbid The presence of two chronic disease or conditions at the same time.

Compounded sterile preparation (CSP) Medication prepared using the sterile compounding processes.

Compounding record (CR) Document (recipe) used to record processes and drugs used to prepare a specific patient's compounded sterile preparation (CSP).

Computerized physician order entry (CPOE) Process of electronic entry of physician orders.

Drug addiction Occurs when attempts to cut back or control use of a controlled substance are unsuccessful.

Drug diversion Any means that deviates the course of a prescription drug from the manufacturer to the intended patient.

Drug misuse Any use of drugs in a manner not directed by a physician.

Drug overdose Injury to the body when a drug is taken in excessive amounts; can be fatal or nonfatal.

Electronic health record (EHR) A patient's complete medical record, including medications and treatment plan; a patient's electronic record that includes health and medication information.

Electronic Medication Administration Record (eMAR) Patient's medication record that is kept electronically.

ExCPT A national exam provided by the National Healthcare Association (NHA) for certification of technicians.

Garbing Donning or putting on personal protective equipment (PPE) in a required series of steps.

Gloved fingertip and thumb sampling Personnel test used to determine whether any microorganisms are present on hands.

Illicit drugs Nonmedical use of a variety of drugs that are prohibited by law, such as cocaine or heroin.

Interdisciplinary care team (ICT) The team approach to treating patients physically, mentally, and spiritually through collaborative efforts of healthcare team members and the patient.

ISO Class 5 area Designated environment for primary engineering control (PEC) used in compounding sterile medications.

ISO Class 7 area Designated area for primary engineering control (PEC) to be kept; also known as a *clean room* or *anteroom.*

ISO Class 8 area Designated area for handwashing and garbing to take place in; also known as a *buffer room.*

Licensure Indicates that an individual has achieved a minimum level of competency.

Master formula record (MFR) A document (recipe) of the processes and medications used in preparing a compounded sterile preparation (CSP).

Media fill testing A test of a prepared compounded sterile preparation (CSP) used to determine the aseptic technique of compounding personnel with the use of a media growth product.

Medication reconciliation Process of creating the most accurate list of medications and treatment notes used in medication adherence programs.

National Association of Boards of Pharmacy (NABP) Nonprofit association that protects public health by assisting its member boards of pharmacy and offers programs that promote safe pharmacy practices for the benefit of consumers.

National Drug Code (NDC) unique 3-segment universal number identifying drug products.

National Healthcare Association (NHA) Organization that offers a certification for pharmacy technicians through the Institute for Certification of Pharmacy Technicians (ICPT).

Opiates Natural opioids such as heroin, morphine, and codeine.

Opioid Natural, semisynthetic, or synthetic opioids.

Opioid use disorder (OUD) Previously known as *drug addiction.*

Patient adherence program Method used for patients to follow medication, treatments, lifestyle, or self-directed regimens in order to stay healthy.

Patient-centered approach A team approach to providing care for patients that includes all parties sharing information and assisting the patient in prevention and ongoing care.

Patient-centered care A team approach to provide care for patients that includes all parties sharing information and assisting the patient in prevention and ongoing care.

Patient-centered model A team approach to provide care for patients that includes all parties sharing information and assisting the patient in prevention and ongoing care.

Periodic automatic replenishment (PAR) level Expected number of items kept on hand at a given time.

Pharmacists' Patient Care Process (PPCP) Developed by The Joint Commission to collaborate with other healthcare providers to provide patient-centered care.

Pharmacogenetics The relationship of how one's genes react to different medications; often interchanged with *pharmacogenomics.*

Pharmacokinetics The study of the movement of drugs throughout the body.

Pharmacy benefits manager (PBM) Controls the submission of claims and any payment to pharmacies as a representative of the insurance company.

Pharmacy Technician Accreditation Council (PTAC) The combination of American Society of Health-System Pharmacists (ASHP) and Accreditation Council for Pharmacy Education (ACPE) to form the accreditation organization for technician training accreditation; accrediting review committee for pharmacy technician education and training programs.

Pharmacy Technician Certification Board (PTCB) Organization that offers national certification of pharmacy technicians (CPhT).

Pharmacy Technician Certification Exam (PTCE) A national exam offered by the Pharmacy Technician Certification Board (PTCB) for certification of technicians.

Point-of-care testing (POCT) As part of the patient-centered approach, early diagnosis and monitoring through tests are used to enhance the patient's overall health.

Point-of-dispensing system (PODS) Temporary area where pharmacy is set up to be point for medication distribution during disasters.

Prescription Drug Monitoring Program (PDMP) State or territorial electronic databases that track controlled substance prescriptions.

Protocol A series of guidelines for a patient to follow that are based on a series of visits or screenings used to achieve a health-related goal.

Radiofrequency identification (RFID) tags Tags used on medications or supplies to transmit data about an item through radio waves to the antenna/reader combination.

Registration Act of maintaining a list of practitioners.

Reimbursement Payment to a provider for services.

Shrinkage inventory loss due to theft or waste.

Standard operating procedure (SOP) Set of procedures used to ensure sterility of all compounded sterile preparations (CSPs).

Sterile Free of living organisms.

Strategic National Stockpile (SNS) National supply of medical and life-saving pharmaceuticals and supplies distributed during disasters.

Surface sampling Test performed to determine whether microorganisms are present on surfaces in the sterile environment areas.

Tiers Levels of responsibilities.

Value-based care System in which payments for services are based on patient outcomes rather than volume; system based on accountability; also known as *accountable care.*

Index

Note: Page numbers followed by *f* indicate figures, *t* indicate tables, and *b* indicate boxes.